Occupational Therapy Administration Manual

Wendy Prabst-Hunt, OTR
President, Courtney Street Rehab Clinic
Rhinelander, Wisconsin and Denver, Colorado

D0207256

DELMAR

THOMSON LEARNING ™

Australia Canada Mexico Singapore Spain United Kingdom United States

DELMAR

THOMSON LEARNING ™

Occupational Therapy Administration Manual
by Wendy Prabst-Hunt

Business Unit Director:
William Brottmiller

Executive Marketing Manager:
Dawn Gerrain

Production Coordinator:
John Mickelbank

Acquisitions Editor:
Candice Janco

Channel Manager:
Gretta Oliver

Art/Design Coordinator
Timothy J. Conners

Editorial Assistant:
Maria D'Angelico

Project Editor:
Mary Ellen Cox

For permission to use material from this text or product, contact us by
Tel   (800) 730-2214
Fax   (800) 730-2215
www.thomsonrights.com

Library of Congress Catalogin-in-Publication Data

Prabst-Hunt, Wendy.
   Occupational therapy administration manual / by Wendy Prabst-Hunt.
      p.. c.m.
   Includes bibliographical references and index.
   ISBN 0–7693–0096–0 (alk. paper)
   1. Occupational therapy -- Management -- Handbooks, manuals, etc. I. Title

RM735.4.P73 2001
615.8'515'068--dc21   2001017226

NOTICE TO THE READER

Publisher does not warrant or guarantee any of the products described herein or perform any independent analysis in connection with any of the product information contained herein. Publisher does not assume, and expressly disclaims, any obligation to obtain and include information other than that provided to it by the manufacturer.

The reader is expressly warned to consider and adopt all safety precautions that might be indicated by the activities herein and to avoid all potential hazards. By following the instructions contained herein, the reader willingly assumes all risks in connection with such instructions.

The Publisher makes no representation or warranties of any kind, including but not limited to, the warranties of fitness for particular purpose or merchantability, nor are any such representations implied with respect to the material set forth herein, and the publisher takes no responsibility with respect to such material. The publisher shall not be liable for any special, consequential, or exemplary damages resulting, in whole or part, from the readers' use of, or reliance upon, this material.

Contents

Preface

The administration of occupational therapy (OT) programs and practices can take on the look of many different practice models. The variety of programs in institutional, community, and private OT departments is infinite. The face of these practice models is transforming in response to reimbursement and legislative changes, and will continue to do so over time.

This textbook was written for the occupational therapist or occupational therapy student who is searching for the tools to effectively manage an OT department or to learn the information necessary to be a leader in the field of OT. It is also appropriate for individuals interested in establishing or expanding a private practice.

For use as an instructional text, case study and discussion questions are included at the end of each chapter. To maximize learning, individuals are encouraged to answer these questions individually or as a group. The reader will find additional information at web addresses and Internet references.

The intention is to bring the reader to a position of understanding about the options for OT programs and methods to be the administrator of a productive and profitable department. It is expected that the reader have knowledge and an understanding of occupational therapy through educational coursework at the undergraduate or graduate level.

Community and alternative program options are among the trends occurring in the field of OT, therefore these are discussed as a method of expanding or establishing new ground for OTs. Resources and management techniques for traditional programs are also addressed in this text; therefore the reader will be able to obtain information appropriate to the operation of many practice settings.

Practical techniques, abundant resources, and Internet links are among the unique aspects of this book. Many suggestions for web interaction will bring the reader within a "click of the mouse" away from additional related information.

The organization of the material can be divided into three sections of the nine total chapters. In the first three chapters, program development, expansion, alternative program options, and private practice issues are covered. This approach allows the reader the opportunity to choose where they are or would like to begin in their journey of OT administration.

The second three chapters move into program implementation. Leadership skills of an OT administrator are discussed as they relate to managing staff. Marketing techniques and promotion of the department, the field of OT, as well as "marketing oneself" are also addressed. Next, the very important issue of reimbursement is offered with links to many resources that will aid the OT administrator in maximizing payment for services.

In the final three chapters, the discussion addresses justifying OT services through appropriate documentation and outcomes research. Technological advances and methods for use in the operations of an OT department are provided.

Because of the tremendous variety of OT practice areas, the differences between regulations in each practice area, and variances between states and reimbursement sources, specific details of each of these topics are not provided. This text is intended to offer the user abundant resources and ways to find the information necessary to carry out the role of program administrator. It is assumed that if an individual is working in a practice setting requiring compliance with specific regulations, the facility or regulating agency will make available the necessary information to the administrator if it is not available here.

It is important to note that this writer and publisher are in no way endorsing any of the products, services, or websites listed in this text. They are simply offered as optional resources for the OT administrator. Web addresses are visually acknowledged in each chapter for ease in retrieval.

Hopefully this resource will guide many to a greater understanding of the rewarding role of OT administrator. By providing the tools to manage in a changing environment, the function of OTs as administrators, private practitioners, and leaders in the field should be maximized.

About the Author

Wendy Prabst-Hunt is a registered occupational therapist and received her bachelors degree from the University of Wisconsin-Milwaukee in 1985. She began her career as a certified occupational therapy assistant in 1981, with an associate degree from Milwaukee Area Technical College. She is a member of Kiwanis International and is a board advisor for the Namlo Foundation, whose mission is to develop programs internationally that guide children and adults to higher education and function.

For the last 14 years, Ms. Prabst-Hunt has been a program developer and occupational therapy manager. She has owned and operated a private occupational therapy practice in northern Wisconsin for six years and is presently expanding services to the Denver, Colorado area. During her career as an OT, Ms. Prabst-Hunt has provided numerous presentations and workshops to her colleagues, and business and industry, within the state of Wisconsin as well as nationally and internationally.

She and her horse offer therapeutic riding to children and adults with special needs in collaboration with Dunroven Farm, Inc. in Rhinelander, Wisconsin. Other personal interests include being with family, travel, mountaineering, and playing handbells at her church. Her professional goals are to continue her education and eventually pursue a career in academia.

Acknowledgments

I would like to express my sincere appreciation to a number of individuals for their professional knowledge, guidance, and expertise. They include Jeanne Plunkett, Barbara Broadbridge, Karen Picus, Margaret Blodgett, Beth Anderson, Jill Mode, Cathy Schelly, and Linda Bolten. Their many contributions have added to the depth of the information provided in this text.

In addition, I would also extend my gratitude to the American Occupational Therapy Association, specifically Marian Scheinholtz, Carla Kieffer, and Heather Hostetler, for their assistance with providing documents, suggestions, and regulatory information necessary to complete this work.

And to my wonderful family and friends, thank you for the encouragement along the way and for always believing in me. Your continual support, kind words, and love will never be forgotten. You all hold a special place in my heart.

CHAPTER 1

Setting Up a New Department

A new occupational therapy (OT) department may be created in a newly opened facility, in an existing setting, or in an established facility that is responding to changes in the health care market. Providing a new service, revising a previous program, and responding to market needs are among the reasons which prompt program initiation.

Meticulous planning is essential to a sound beginning for any developing OT department. Advanced preparation provides the foundation for a quality program with potential for future growth and expansion. In each scenario, an OT manager will need to respond to opportunities and identify areas of need.

Clear goals, a strategic plan, and a mission guide the OT manager in projecting the type of service, budget, staffing, space, and equipment needs of the program. A stable department requires committed employees; therefore, the ability to recruit and retain staff becomes paramount. These issues constitute the building blocks for this challenging but rewarding task and will be discussed further in this chapter.

At the conclusion of this chapter, the reader will be able to:

1. Identify reasons for opening a new department and analyze its competition.

2. Write a mission statement for a developing practice.

3. Determine staffing needs; understand the recruitment, interview, and hiring process.

4. Identify equipment needs for a new occupational therapy department.

5. Understand the essentials of financial planning for an OT department.

Strategic Planning, Goals, Missions, and Visions

The development of a strategic plan is the basis for a new program and for the continuation of future services. A department created without a plan will lack direction and focus. Beginning with a set vision, the OT manager may address the following questions with strategic management (Solomon, 1991):

- What is the relationship of the program to society? (i.e., mission statement)

- How will this program serve its community?

- What is the intended role of this department in several years?

- What changes may occur in health care delivery, the consumer population to be served, competing services, or trends in the community that may affect this program in the future?
- What preparations must be made to address the possible obstacles to the future success of this program?

Strategic planning is completed when the following steps are taken, according to Hillestad and Berkowitz (1991):

- Define the area of practice.
- Identify competitors.
- Determine differences among competitors.
- Forecast environmental change.

However, Solomon describes the process of a strategic plan as *planning* and *implementation*. He further states that planning: defines the mission of a department, translates the mission into long- and short-term objectives, and develops a strategy for achieving those goals. Implementation, then, is putting the plan into action.

Schultz and Johnson (1990) recommend completing the strategic planning process in a participatory, facilitative manner, which involves gathering input from staff within the department, but may extend to eliciting feedback from sources within the rest of the facility and in the community. This approach helps to gain the perspective of staff, other departments, or community resources, which can add positive building blocks for growth.

Developing a Mission Statement

The mission statement assists in defining an area of practice. Included in the mission statement is the intent of the department, the population it proposes to serve, the age groups of its intended population, the specific service that it will provide, any geographical location information which may be pertinent, treatment philosophies, and the department's attitude toward service. In other words, the mission statement defines what is of primary importance to the department (Schultz and Johnson, 1990). For example, of importance to the program or practice may be quality, experience, and friendliness, to name a few. See Figure 1.1 for Sample Mission Statement.

Identifying Strengths, Weaknesses, Opportunities, Threats

Solomon (1991) suggests preparation of a SWOT analysis (SWOT is an acronym for strength, weakness, opportunities, and threats) as another of the strategic planning stages. An effective strategy will build upon strengths, compensate for weaknesses, capitalize on opportunities, and defend against threats.

Anticipate potential barriers and challenges early in development. By asking "What can prevent the department from reaching its goals?" and "How can the department respond to changes in the health care arena?" the program will

---

The mission of MVRC is to provide high quality pediatric occupational therapy to children ages birth to 21, in their natural environment, throughout the communities of Summit and Lakeview Counties.

Figure 1.1 Sample Mission Statement

be braced to respond appropriately when the need arises. Refer to Figure 1.2 for a Sample SWOT Analysis.

Defining the Competition

It is important to examine competing services when planning a new program. Solomon (1991) recommends using a "competitive analysis." This requires determining overlap, duplication, or gaps in services provided. Identify the direct and indirect competition. Understand their strengths and weaknesses by asking some pertinent questions such as:

- Who is the competition?
- Are there duplications in services provided?
- What is the potential for new competition?
- Is the market growing, diminishing, or steady?
- How is the proposed program different from others in the same geographical area?

Goal Setting

Goal setting is an important, ongoing process in the OT department. Short-term goals (STG) address issues to be completed within six months to one year.

STRENGTHS

1. Location
2. Experience
3. Reputation
4. Motivated therapist
5. Stable staff
6. Atmosphere

WEAKNESSES

1. High profile competition
2. Relatively small budget
3. Small clinic (can also be a strength)
4. Minimal time to market services
5. Therapist often going many directions
6. Office isn't always "open"

OPPORTUNITIES

1. Growth potential
2. Possibility for additional contracts
3. Market need for occupational therapy services in birth to three programs in neighboring counties
4. Many marketing opportunities in neighboring communities

THREATS

1. Large facility competition
2. Change in regulations for payment of OT services in the future?
3. Large employer's potential change of group insurance to carrier in a non-participating plan
4. Continued reductions in government insurance reimbursement for OT services
5. Referral sources leaving the area

BARRIERS (to reaching full potential) – optional

1. Poor motivation to schedule physician visits, physician/marketing visits
2. Manager frequently out of the office
3. Fluctuating "in" office hours due to multi-location services

---

Figure 1.2   Sample SWOT Analysis

Long-term goals (LTG) are used to keep a department focused on progress and growth over a more extended period of time. LTGs may contain three to five year projections. Goal setting is helpful for program implementation as well as for budgeting, staff development, and for program growth.

Employees should be asked to identify individual professional goals. Attempting to coordinate staff goals with department projections can empower strengths and encourage professional development. Ongoing communication about department and professional employee goals will aid in cohesion, stability, and natural growth of the department.

Schultz and Johnson (1990) address a number of important criteria for effective long range planning:

- Plans should be based on a thorough study of the needs of the organization.

- Broad participation is needed to increase effective planning and implementation of the plans. In addition to consumers, whose participation can be accomplished through personal, phone, or group contact, medical staff and other pertinent employees should be included.

- Plans should be comprehensive.

The effectiveness of the strategic plan should be evaluated biannually to annually. This is done by reevaluating present goals for appropriateness. Revising goals and the plan as indicated encourages stability and future growth.

Looking Ahead

Forecasting environmental change, as earlier recommended by Hillestad and Berkowitz (1991), is an element of strategic planning. Being aware of possible legislative changes, reimbursement or staffing trends, plans by the competition to expand, and new business intentions enables an organization to prepare in advance for change.

Space Requirements and Square Footage Needs

The space and square footage needs of an office will be directly correlated to issues of number of staff, type of treatment performed, and anticipated amount of space usage. Consider each of the points below when justifying amount of space required. The number of staff currently and expected in 3 to 5 years, types of treatment planned and aspired for in the future, anticipated space usage now and later (estimated units per day per room), and population served all have a significant impact on the type and amount of space needed. Accessibility requirements of the Americans with Disabilities Act (ADA) and Medicare must also be considered. The ADA can be accessed at www.usdoj.gov/crt/ada/adahom1.htm or and outlines accessibility guidelines. AOTA president, Barbara Kornbleau, also has a very informative website for the occupational therapist. It not only provides accessibility information, but also gives the OT manager legal, legislative, governmental, health policy, ethical, and lobbying links and resources. To visit this website go to: http://www.nova.edu/~kornblau/index.html.

Hosford-Dunn, Dunn, and Harford, (1995) recommend the comfort of the space be evaluated by using the checklist below:

- Interior lighting (adequate for treatment, soft for relaxation)

- Exterior lighting for safe evening appointments
- Colors and ambiance (consumer comfort and ease, professional appearance)
- Layout of rooms (easy access between rooms and ability to dovetail treatment sessions when appropriate)
- Music/noise (noise level between rooms, background music)
- Restrooms/drinking fountain (availability, conveniently located)
- Kitchen facilities (refrigerator, microwave, sink, lounge)
- Location (professional district, conveniently located, parking easy to find and accessible)
- Building construction (safe environment for staff and consumers)
- Signs (clearly displayed, limited confusion)

Department square footage can be categorized as clinic space, offices, reception and waiting room, restrooms, lounge, and storage. If the space is limited, questions that address space allocation are:

- Can any of these rooms overlap?
- Could therapist desk be incorporated into clinic space?
- Can the lounge/break area be part of the activities of daily living (ADL) kitchen?
- Are separate rooms needed for office/reception staff and waiting area?
- Can rooms be subdivided?
- Is there room for expansion?

Planning for Expansion

The type of space and amount of square footage needed should be reflected in the department goals. When planning to add therapists, office staff, treatment programs, and/or equipment, it is appropriate to acquire space or identify opportunities for remodeling and expansion initially. A thriving department rarely remains constant during the first five years, although eventually a plateau will occur. Inadequate space until that time inhibits department growth and potential. Therefore, if these preparations are made initially, future expansions will become a natural transition.

Clinic Space. Clinic space can be divided into individual treatment rooms and group treatment areas. Individual rooms should be a minimum of approximately 10 ft. X 10 ft. to accommodate a total of one to three people. Large clinic areas can be used for group therapy or to house several treatment tables. Many consumers can be accommodated simultaneously within a large treatment room. If possible, subdivide or assign separate rooms for pediatrics and meal preparation.

Curtained or private treatment areas should always be offered for soft tissue work, myofascial release treatments, severe trauma situations, and self-cares. Individual treatment rooms are necessary for biofeedback, psychological inter- and intrapersonal services, and therapeutic massage.

If pediatric treatment is planned, hanging equipment securely from the ceiling using hooks and net storage will eliminate unsafe clutter and reduce distractions.

For group therapy or meeting rooms, a warm, secure, and comfortable atmosphere is critical to aid the group process. The rooms should invite open expression of thoughts and feelings. Clinical rooms should have a clean and professional appearance without projecting a bare, cold feeling. Prints or photographs on the walls and the availability of interesting or educational material help create a competent yet relaxed ambiance.

Office and Reception Area. A primary consideration for office space is confidentiality. Consumer information should not be available (visually or auditorally) within the office. Therefore, if treatment rooms are combined with therapist/office space, dictation and phone calls need to be done when consumers are not immediately present. Similarly, charts and other consumer information need to be covered or filed. The above rules also apply to office staff if this space is combined with the waiting area. Schedules, bills, and medical records should not be displayed in any way to the casual view of the public. Telephone business, including confidential information, must be completed quietly and privately.

Whether private or group offices are used, an attempt at efficiency and organization will prevent unnecessary frustration and loss of productivity. Cabinet, book, and file storage, copy machine, fax, telephone, and computer should be arranged with work simplification and ergonomic considerations. Built-in casework or modular areas, as opposed to freestanding desks, can provide for efficient use of space and may offer customized storage for many supplies and types of equipment.

Restrooms. Restrooms for consumers and staff are best located on the same floor and close to treatment and reception areas. Ample facilities are necessary and will depend on consumer volume and staff size. Grab bar placement, door width, sink and paper towel height, faucet and door handle type, and force needed to operate are among those restroom characteristics to consider when making choices for new construction or renovation. This information can be found by looking at the Title III Regulation: Public Accommodations and Services operated by Private Entities, Part 36 and at the ADA Accessibility Guidelines (ADAAG) on the ADA home page at www.usdoj.gov/crt/ada/adahom1.htm.

Storage Rooms. A storage room will be beneficial only if it is large enough. Without proper space or room for organization, retrieving items can be burdensome and very time consuming. Often, a "stacking" or "cramming" technique is popular in these situations, which refers to the chronological order of items placed there, i.e., the first item is placed on the bottom or in the back and the last item is placed on the top or in the front. When attempting to obtain an item on the bottom, severe inconvenience occurs. This creates unnecessarily wasted time and irritation. Also, if large items (wheelchair, infrequently used equipment, portable evaluation kits, etc.) are stored in close proximity, there is a tendency for larger items to become stacked in front of the shelves and files as items accumulate. This will cause the same inconvenience as previously mentioned.

Shelving and filing helps this situation. To avoid these pitfalls in use of storage space, it is helpful to subdivide storage space or design more than one location for storage initially. For example, large equipment and paper supplies should be stored separately.

Lounge/Break Area. In some cases, it might be necessary to have a "break" room. Other rooms such as personnel offices, ADL kitchen, or aid station may suffice. If these rooms are used for staff breaks and lunch, it remains imperative that confidentiality is upheld as it relates to consumer information. In addition, consumers should not have to listen to the latest gossip or weekend events discussed between staff due to location of this break area.

Employees need to have uninterrupted break and lunch opportunities. Therefore policies regarding responding to work, phone calls, or messages should be enforced. Employees should be encouraged to leave the work area for lunch and breaks. Break rooms often contain a microwave, refrigerator, and sink for lunch storage and preparation. If an activities of daily living (ADL) kitchen exists, this area can house these amenities. However, staff lunches need to be kept separate from consumer supplies. In this situation, a break room would be helpful. A table and chairs are integral; a couch is a bonus. If space is limited, alternating lunch hours between staff could solve the problem.

Waiting Room. The waiting room is usually the first impression the consumer has of the rehabilitation or OT department. The consumer may be nervous, upset, afraid, guarded, or in a hurry. He/she needs to feel at ease upon arriving in the department. The waiting room should offer soft lighting for reading, offering a calm atmosphere. Enough comfortable seating should be used to accommodate present as well as incoming appointments. Colors and decorating style should be pleasant and light. Provide appropriate reading material to ease waiting time. Books and toys for children should be available for entertainment and to help avoid waiting room disruptions. Coffee is optional, but access to water is important.

The receptionist needs to be efficient, friendly, and compassionate. Assistance should be offered in a timely manner without giving the impression of being inconvenienced. Office staff should offer individual guidance for paperwork, if the consumer is unable to complete it independently for any reason. Bringing consumers to their designated treatment rooms on schedule, even if a further wait is expected, alleviates space problems in waiting rooms and makes a consumer feel attended to.

Accreditation and Survey Compliance

There are several governing agencies that accredit health care facilities, and OT is included in the compliance standards, which require an on-site survey periodically. The purpose of becoming accredited or certified by these agencies is to validate the reputation of the facility or program, facilitate ease in reimbursement, and assure positive outcomes of medical care. Because these credentialling agencies focus on quality of care, the facility's benefit from this rigorous process is to ensure that high quality programs and procedures are in place. Upon successful survey results, the facility may realize a positive community perception from this status. The Joint Commission on Accreditation of Healthcare Organizations (JCAHO), the Commission on Accreditation of Rehabilitation Facilities (CARF), and Medicare are among those credentialling agencies used for Occupational Therapy programs.

JCAHO accredits hospitals, health care networks, long term care facilities, ambulatory care facilities, home care organizations, clinical laboratories, and behavioral health care facilities. Standards are rigorous and address the organizations' level of performance for activities that affect the quality of care while aiming to improve outcomes. Each department within the facility has its own set of standards and guidelines. The latest versions of the standards are published in comprehensive accreditation manuals for each accreditation program, and include scoring guidelines. To order a copy of the accreditation manual or more information on JCAHO, visit www.jcaho.org/accred/.

CARF is an accrediting agency for adult day service, assisted living, behavioral health, employment and community services, and medical rehabilitation. The organization promotes quality, value, and optimal outcomes through its accreditation process. To prepare for a CARF survey, CARF recommends purchasing the manual specific to the service or organization. CARF offers two manuals for each area: the *Standards Manual* and the *Survey Preparation Guide*. To obtain further information, go to www.carf.org.

Medicare surveys are performed for new clinics and programs when Medicare certification is requested. An application process is completed to obtain a group and or individual provider number and in some cases an on-site visit is required. To obtain information about survey guidelines for Medicare state to state, contact the Medicare fiscal intermediary listed in Figure 7.1, p. 114.

Staffing and Employment

The management of personnel can be one of the most difficult albeit rewarding aspects of the position of OT manager. It requires careful consideration to caseload, trends, and personalities, while juggling budget constraints with salaries and benefits. Program growth requires stable staff, which translates into positive recruitment and retention practices.

Recruitment

When additional staff becomes necessary to meet program demands, recruitment and retention emerge as critical issues in the operation of the department. Targeting the "right person for the job" is of primary importance, and should not be overlooked in lieu of a "quick hire" to fill the vacancy. Although the recruitment and hiring process is often time consuming, waiting for a good match between employee and employer will save time and money over time.

When carrying a full patient caseload or operating short staffed, finding time for the recruitment process is often difficult. In many facilities, the human resources department is available to do many of the tasks involved in hiring employees. However, if you are the primary person to perform this sometimes-arduous job, the timeline becomes a concern. A minimum of one to two months is necessary at times to recruit a therapist. Additional time is sometimes required if an individual is relocating. Filling office or paraprofessional staff positions demands training until learning and confidence increase. Therefore, planning ahead is beneficial. Keep a file of resumes and inquiries received, for future reference. Interns should be encouraged to submit a resume upon completion of clinical fieldwork. In addition, during recruitment periods, having a list of therapists willing to provide temporary fill-in work is helpful, to avoid burning out the current staff.

Before beginning the hiring process, identify the skills required of the employee. For instance:

- Is it necessary to find an occupational therapy assistant (OTA) with experience in pediatrics?
- Does this position require the expertise of a certified hand therapist (CHT)?
- Can this position be filled with a new graduate?
- Would an experienced OT better fill the need of the OT department?
- Is experience in a specific area of practice required?

An applicant should have at least some exposure to and more than a passing interest in learning about the area of practice in question, even if an entry-level therapist is considered. Previous students make excellent candidates for vacant positions because they come with knowledge of daily operations. Reviewing the role delineation for OTs and OTAs will define the differences in responsibilities between the two positions. It is important to review the position of any applicable state certification or licensure agency and the AOTA's official position when determining if an opening should be filled with an OT or OTA.

The documents supporting the delineation of roles between occupational therapists and occupational therapy assistants are being reviewed within the American Occupational Therapy Association. The AOTA's current position is the "Occupational Therapy Roles," AOTA 2000, which rescinded the "Entry Level Role Delineation for Registered Occupational Therapists (OTs) and Certified Occupational Therapy Assistants (OTAs), AOTA 1981." However, a new paper entitled "Skill Mix Paper" has been written and posted at www.aota.org to increase the ease in clarifying the roles between therapists. Appendix 1.1 presents the current AOTA position, but the reader is also referred to the other two documents.

Clarifying Position Vacancies

After the positions have been approved, the next step is to determine the salary range and benefit package to be offered. Outline additional perks of the job such as flexible time and continuing education. Will a sign-on bonus be included? Will relocation assistance or interview expenses be provided?

The supply and demand for OT staff will dictate the extent to which some benefits are demanded. In a market where OTs are limited and in great demand, sign-on bonuses for example are often required. However, when the job market is saturated with OTs these additional benefits may not be necessary.

Advertising for Vacancies

Next, decide what avenues will be used to begin the recruitment process. The cost of advertising may influence the choices. Knowing where a population of OT recruits may exist will influence the decision about where ads will be placed. Consideration about relocation must be given if choosing to run ads in national publications or on the internet.

Some options for finding applicants for position vacancies include buut are not limited to:

1. Word of mouth. Let colleagues know of open positions. Be careful of interterritorial conflicts, however.
2. Local area newspapers
3. State association newsletters
4. Professional journals
5. National, state, and local OT meetings or continuing education opportunities.
6. Recruitment agencies
7. Internet postings
8. Direct or bulk mailing
9. Job fairs
10. On-campus recruiting or advertising

Program Promotion

After the the position(s) have been filled, the next step is to determine where to begin advertising. Here are some suggestions:

1. Word of mouth. Let colleagues know of open positions (be careful of interterritorial conflicts however).

2. Local area newspapers.

3. State association newsletters.

4. OT journals.

5. Recruitment agencies.

Determine the salary range and benefit package to be offered. Outline additional perks of the job such as flexible time and continuing education. Will a sign-on bonus be included? Will relocation assistance or interview expenses be provided?

The supply and demand for OT staff will dictate the extent to which some benefits are demanded. In a market when OTs are limited and in great demand, sign-on bonuses for example are often required. However, when the job market is saturated with OTs, these additional benefits may not be necessary.

Reviewing a Resume

The process of selecting a new employee begins with reviewing a resume and cover letter. For the employer, these documents serve to screen all applicants based on qualifications and compatibility to the position. The resume provides a screening process for the interview potential of the candidate (Lore, 1999). If the applicant positively conveys why they are the right person for the job, then they may be worth considering for an interview. When reviewing a resume or cover letter, confirm that the applicant meets educational and experience requirements, projects a professional image through written work (grammar, spelling, and writing), and offers references. Timelines for education and employment that contain gaps should be questioned.

Reviewing resumes typically helps to reduce the number of face-to-face interviews required to fill an open position. However, in areas where OT/OTA shortages exist, the manager is advised to continue interviewing even after the initial vacancy is filled. The manager should be honest that the interview is for *future* openings.

The Interview Process

Some of the following information was posted by the University of Kansas Department of Communication Studies at their web site: http://www.ukans.edu/cwis/units/coms2/via/planning2.html and contains some material from "Effective Interviewing," Down, Cal W., Harper & Row, Inc.

After reviewing the resumes received, the manager must make decisions about the employment potential of the applicants. If interested in pursuing a candidate, the manager's next step is to set up the interview. Planning the interview process in advance will greatly increase the effectiveness of the interview.

Setting up the Interview

Before contacting the applicant, decide the purpose and direction of the interview. Be prepared. These issues are among those to discuss during the initial conversation:

- The position available; number of hours, type of consumer, size of staff and facility.
- Candidate's level of interest in interviewing for the position.
- *When* position is available.
- Availability of the applicant.

When setting up the interview, offering flexibility in meeting times, i.e., evenings and weekends, may assist the applicant with scheduling and create a positive first impression of the employer. On the other hand, inflexibility in scheduling may have a negative impact, which can carry over into future interactions.

There are times when the interview is conducted for purposes of general information gathering and simply to meet the candidate and, for example, to establish future resources. This should be communicated openly during the initial telephone contact, as previously mentioned.

Planning for the Interview

Because the interview is used to obtain more information about the applicant, consider the elements of primary interest and design the questions accordingly. Consistency must be applied to all applicants during the interview process. Law prohibits use of questions regarding age, marital status, race, religion, childcare, transportation, or disability (Hosford-Dunn, Dunn, and Harford, 1995 and Kishel and Kishel, 1993). Some areas to review may be:

- Quality of experience and expertise.
- Special interest areas.
- Expectations of a job.
- Expectations of a supervisor.
- Strengths and areas for improvement.
- Likes and dislikes of present position.
- Methods of handling workplace conflict.
- Future (one to five year) professional goals.
- Level of organization.
- Level of motivation for growth.
- Ideas about position applied for.
- Handling of negative feedback and criticism.
- Level of compatibility with present position.

Formulating Interview Questions

In the "pre-offer" stage of the interview, the Americans with Disabilities Act (ADA) regulates the types of questions that can be asked related to disabilities. At this stage the employer cannot ask questions that are likely to elicit information about a disability. This includes directly asking whether an applicant has a particular disability. Appendix A-1.4, ADA Guidelines to Disability–Related

Questions, answers some commonly asked questions about this area of the law. This and other ADA documents can be obtained free of charge at www.usdoj. gov/crt/ada/qandaeng.htm.

In formulating questions for the interview, identify those areas of primary importance, while considering acceptable and unacceptable questions. Use open-ended questions. In Figure 1.3 Hosford-Dunn, et al. provide guidelines regarding discriminatory interview questions. Figure 1.4 offers suggestions for interview questions that may be used by the OT manager.

Conducting the Interview

Being prepared for the interview will increase its success. Plan the physical setting of the interview and where the meeting will occur. Avoid sitting behind a

ACCEPTABLE QUESTIONS	UNACCEPTABLE QUESTIONS
Have you ever used another name?	What is your maiden name?
What is your place of residence?	Do you own or rent your own home?
Are you over 18 years old?	What is your birth date?
Can you provide verification of your right to work in the U.S.?	Are you a U.S. citizen?
What languages can you speak, read or write?	Where were you born?
	What is your native tongue?
	Where were your parents born?
Can you perform the functions of this job with or without reasonable accommodation?	Do you have any physical disabilities?
How would you perform these functions?	Do you have a disability that would interfere in your ability to perform the job?
Can you meet the attendance requirements of this job?	How many days were you sick last year?
Have you ever been convicted of a felony?	Have you ever been arrested?
What skills have you acquired through military service?	When did you serve in the military?
	How were you discharged?
What professional organizations you do you belong to?	What organizations or clubs do belong to?
	What is your height and weight?
	What race are you?
	What does your spouse do?
	How many children do you have?
	How old are your children?

Figure 1.3   Guidelines Regarding Discriminatory Questions (Hosford-Dunn, Dunn, and Harford, 1995)

- How would you describe your clinical skills?
- What are your favorite areas of practice?
- What do you like best about being an OT/COTA/office manager, etc.?
- What do you like the least?
- Describe what expectations you have for your next job.
- Describe the qualities you would like to see in your next supervisor.
- Explain what you believe to be your strengths.
- What do others see as your strengths?
- What areas do you feel you need to improve?
- What have others given you constructive feedback about?
- How do you handle workplace conflict?
- Describe your reaction to constructive feedback or criticism.
- How do you feel you would meet the needs of the present opening?
- What ideas do you have about the position?
- What new areas of practice would you like to learn?
- List short and long range goals for yourself.
- How timely are you with deadlines and paperwork requirements?
- Can you perform the functions of this job with or without reasonable accommodations?

Figure 1.4   Appropriate Interview Questions

desk to conduct the interview. If there are other individuals who will join the meeting, determine when this will occur. If the applicant is to be taken to another location to meet with co-workers or supervisors, schedule this and a tour of the facility into the plan. It is also appropriate to arrange brief contact with consumers, as indicated. Observations of interaction between the interviewee and consumers may provide valuable information about the compatibility of the applicant to the job.

Lore (1999) describes using a clearly written agenda that will guide the manager and facilitate the flow of the meeting. Although the applicant should do 80 percent of the talking, it is the responsibility of the OT manager to set the course of the meeting. An example of an interview agenda may be as follows:

- Clearly reiterate the purpose of the meeting and the position applied for.
- Communicate anticipated schedule and process of interview.
- Describe position in detail and give job description.
- Be honest about challenges as well as positive aspects of the position.
- Discuss expectations for an individual in this role.
- Explain the needs of the department as they relate to the vacancy.
- Begin questioning.
- Meet with pertinent co-workers.
- Meet OT staff.
- Tour facility.
- Regroup for final questions and answers.
- Closure. A positive closure to the meeting is one that leaves the applicant and interviewer with an understanding of what is to happen next.

Making the Right Choice

With more than one applicant, choosing the best match for the job becomes a necessity. A successful interview should provide enough information to help make this decision. Obtaining feedback from others involved in the interview process is helpful, but ultimately the OT manager has the final responsibility for the decision. Using a list of "pros" and "cons" can be helpful in making difficult choices.

Neither employer nor employee should enter into relocation to a new or unfamiliar geographical location lightly. Reasons for relocation need attention, as well as whether the location can meet the needs of all parties involved.

The professional goals of the applicant should be compatible with the future plans of the department. A potential employee with no interest in pediatrics may not be a candidate for an OT department that plans to expand to the school district, even if it may not occur for a year or two.

The right person for the job will:

- Enjoy doing the work applied for.
- Excel at required job skills.
- Have career goals that are compatible to the job description and department needs.
- Convey a positive self-image.
- Will raise no "red flags" for the interviewer. (Red flags are those behaviors or responses that spark a negative or uneasy feeling in the interviewer.)

Check references with previous employers. Do not overlook concerns, as they will later return to cause problems in the department if ignored.

When a decision has been made, make an offer of employment to the chosen individual. If the candidate accepts, contact the remaining applicants (by written correspondence or telephone) to notify them of the decision. If the offer is not accepted, continue the negotiation process and/or make an offer to the second choice candidate. A written followup regarding the offer is recommended.

Establish a start date, hours, and appropriate dress. Develop a training schedule. Each employee will require a different level of training and supervision to become independent as a therapist. The OT manager must work with the employee to establish a comfort level on the job before requiring complete autonomy in the position. Document all orientation and training to reduce legal risks. Use of a flow sheet verifying information instructed in orientation, which the employee and employer both sign, is a good method of recording new employee training sessions.

Equipment Needs for a New Department

Equipment needs are divided into two categories: *capital* and *operational*. Capital expenses are those in which the purchase price of the item received is over a specified dollar amount, e.g., over $500.00. These are pieces of equipment that will be used for a longer period of time (i.e., two years minimum). A fluidotherapy unit, computer equipment, or staff desks are examples of capital equipment purchases. Operating supplies are those which are replaced regularly and cost under approximately $500.00 (differs based on facility policy). These include items such as patient and office supplies, small equipment, assistive devices, and splinting tools.

There are two primary department needs in terms of capital furniture and equipment: office and clinical. A third need for some facilities may be characterized as mobile equipment. This category may be necessary for separation in some cases when outreach services are supplied.

Office and Clinic Equipment

Facilities that have in-house billing and transcription departments will have many of their clerical needs met. A centralized receptionist may do the scheduling for OT as well as physical therapy (PT) and speech pathology. Freestanding OT clinics will have greater needs in the area of office equipment because they need to coordinate transcription, billing, and reception. The types of office and clinic equipment required in nontraditional settings will vary greatly, depending on facility and consumer needs. Every setting, however, will require some office, clerical, and therapeutic supplies, equipment, and resources in order to carry out every day functions in support of the clinicians. A sample equipment and supply list is provided in Figure 1.5.

Budgeting

The value of creating an OT budget is in its potential for supplying future information useful for financial planning (Jacobs & Logigian, 1999 and Bangs, 1998a). Figures should be calculated for monthly and annual projections, based on the fiscal year used (e.g., January 1st to December 31st). A three-year projection also provides future direction and promotes vision. The result is a tool to guide the OT manager in monitoring the financial aspects of the department.

Documents Associated with the Budget Process

There are several components of the budget process. The capital budget, operational budget, and monthly projections are among the primary financial documents written by the occupational therapy manager.

Capital Budget. Those items and building charges which exceed a specified dollar amount, e.g., $500.00. The length of use for capital purchases should be at least two to three years. These items are calculated for depreciation and, therefore, tax benefits may be available. Computer equipment, for example, constitutes a capital purchase. Justifications are generally required by facilities for purchasing capital items. To justify a requested purchase, provide reasons of necessity and expected revenue increases as a result of the item.

Operational Budget. This represents the daily operations of the department, from salaries to patient supplies. It includes information about revenues (income generated), and type and number of personnel (full or part-time, positions held).

Monthly Projections. This is the part of the operations budget which identifies fluctuations in revenue and expenses. Rationalization for trends are provided, e.g., planned continuing education, expected increase in salaries, increase or decrease in revenues with school year contracts, etc.

Monthly Comparisons. Compiling a "days adjusted basis" report compares the number of days in the month to the revenues and expenses. For instance, March may appear to have greater revenues than February, but the number of business days per month is likely to be different. What is the average profit realized per workday each month?

SWOT Analysis. Strategic planning can be associated with budgeting or included separately in departmental planning. For more information about SWOT analysis, see page 2 and Figure 1.2.

CAPITAL OFFICE EQUIPMENT

Computer equipment
Personal computer(s)
Printer(s)
Optional/scanner, projector
Laptop
Software, billing, scheduling, presentation
Copier
Telephone system
Fax
Intercom
Overhead music
Desks, freestanding or built-in files, cabinets, tablesDesk tools
Desk chairs
Side chairs

OPERATING OFFICE SUPPLIES

Magazines/holder
Newspapers
Brochures
Plants & decorations (optional)
Pens/paper and supplies
File folders
Business cards
Copier maintenance
Toner, etc.
Disks
Stapler
Stack trays

CAPITAL CLINIC EQUIPMENT
(Dependent on area of practice)

Furniture
Clinic/group tables
Mat tables
Chairs, side, wheeled

Exercise Equipment
Pulleys
Work stimulation
Pediatric balls, bolsters, swings
Weights and storage
Recreation tools, bowling alley, mini-golf
Therapeutic pool, jungle gym

Modalities
Fluidotherapy
Paraffin
Refrigerator/freezer
Hydroculator
Iontophoresis

Neuromuscular electrical stimulation
TENS

Biofeedback
Upper-extremity whirlpool
Mobile splint cart

ADL Supplies
Kitchen
Bathroom
Washer/dryer
Work simulation devices
Driving evaluation tools (rarely seen in occupational therapy departments)
Tools and woodworking supplies
Greenhouse or horticulture therapy (raised garden bed)
Computer and educational/clinical software

Figure 1.5   Equipment and Supply List *(continues)*

OPERATING CLINIC SUPPLIES

Therapy Tools

Play-doh

Hand grippers

Theraband

Weights

Manual dexterity tools

ADLs

Adaptive equipment

Food

Garden supplies

Wood supplies

Paper and writing tools

Clothing or dressing boards

Relaxation tapes

Paint

Soap

Sport equipment, balls and games

Craft supplies, assistive technology devices

Positioning devices

Ergonomic tools

Modality/Medical

Electrodes

Gels

Towels

Gloves

Dressing/wound care supplies

Splint pan

Gowns

Fluidotherapy refill

Splints

Other

Reference Books

Some evaluation tools/supplies

CAPITAL MOBILE EQUIPMENT
(Variable based on services provided; outreach vs. outstation)

Automobile (may choose to pay mileage instead of purchasing)

Cell phone

Evaluation kits

Dictaphone

Computer, laptop

Fax

Copier

Computer software, including Internet, scheduling, network

OPERATING MOBILE EQUIPMENT

Exercise equipment

Treatment devices

General office supplies

Suitcase, tote bag, carrier

Figure 1.5   Equipment and Supply List *(continued)*

Expenses and Revenues

The budget process for a newly established department begins with identifying *estimated* expenses and revenues, and creating the budget proposal. Because no financial history exists, compiling this data can be a challenge. However even a long-standing practice should occasionally revert to "zero-based budgeting" (vs. historic budgeting) to fully understand expense control. Zero-based budgeting examines an expense from the previous year beginning with zero (instead of adding costs to the budget automatically from year to year). If each expense is justified for actual need in this way, control of expenses is maintained.

Expenses. Determine costs for fixed expenses first. Rent, lease purchases, and loan payments may be among those items which remain constant each month. For instance, if a piece of equipment is being leased for $150.00 a month, the annual budgeted amount is $1,800.00 and this expense will remain the same for the length of the lease (e.g., 24 months).

Variable Expenses. Variable expenses can then be projected by estimating costs of items such as telephone, utilities, office supplies, advertising, dues and subscriptions, travel/education, taxes, salaries, insurance, meals and entertainment, and charitable contributions. Depreciation is a non-cash expense calculated by an accountant for purposes of tax credits. Client and civic relations, bank charges, repairs and maintenance, postage, and laundry can also be given separate line items to more clearly delineate expenses.

Revenues. Projected revenues (or income generated) are calculated by creating some assumptions. For example:

1. One person working 40 hours per week (8 hours per day) will be able to generate a predetermined number of treatment units, otherwise known as productive time or productivity.

2. Standard estimated productivity, e.g., 60 percent of the workday is spent generating billable treatment units. Eight hours per day at 60 percent productivity equals approximately 5 hours or 20 quarter-hour units per day of billable time.

3. Volume or caseload is substantial enough to meet 60 percent productivity for approximately 48 weeks per year.

4. A percentage of units billed will not be collected due to discounted insurance rates, Medicare and Medicaid denials/caps, bad debt, etc. Setting a goal to collect 80 percent of all charges, for example, will assist the billing process and set targets for future change if needed.

5. Twenty units per day X the average cost of treatment unit (i.e., $40.00) equals $800.00 X 80 percent actual reimbursement equals $640.00 revenue per day worked or $3,200.00 per week, for a 5-day week.

6. Staff with 2 weeks vacation, continuing education, and sick time will be productive for approximately 48 weeks per year.

7. One full time equivalent (FTE) person has potential to generate $153,600.00 actual revenue per year, depending on available caseload.

Following the development and implementation of a budget proposal, and after the budget becomes operational, actual ongoing financial reports are compiled. A monthly, quarterly, and annual income statement, otherwise known as a profit and loss statement (P & L) (Figure 1.6) is supplied by an accountant or computer program based on income received and expenses incurred each month. The P & L *does not* record outstanding revenues generat-

CURRENT, YTD, AND RATIOS				
	Current	%	Year-to-Date	%
Income				
Service Income	17,000.00	85.0	175,000.00	
Patient Fees	3,000.00	15.0	28,000.00	
Fee Refunds	-0-		-3,000.00	
Total Income	20,000.00	100.0	200,000.00	100.0
Cost of Goods Sold				
Subcontractor #1	500.00	5.0	1,000.00	0.3
Subcontractor #2	0.00	0	500.00	0.2
Total Cost of Sales	500.00	5.0	1,50.00	0.5
Gross Profit (Loss)	19,500.00	95.0	198,500.00	95.0
Expenses				
Payroll	8,000.00	61.0	96,000.00	65.0
Advertising	200.00	1.5	1,200.00	0.8
Office Supplies	100.00	1.0	600.00	0.4
Travel	300.00	2.0	1,500.00	1.0
Education/Seminars	300.00	2.0	1,000.00	0.7
Operating Supplies	500.00	4.0	6,000.00	4.0
Insurance	200.00	1.5	700.00	0.5
Rent Expense	500.00	4.0	6,000.00	4.0
Accounting	100.00	1.0	1,200.00	0.8
Taxes	2,400.00	18.0	30,000.00	20.0
Telephone	200.00	1.5	1,200.00	0.8
Dues & Subscriptions	50.00	0.04	600.00	0.4
Bank Charges	10.00	0.01	120.00	0.08
Laundry	50.00	0.05	600.00	0.4
Depreciation Expense	200.00	1.5	1,200.00	0.8
Total Expenses	13,060.00	67.0	147,920.00	74.5
Operating Income (Loss)	6,440.00	33.0	50,580.00	25.5
Other Income				
Interest Income	60.00	0.3	420.00	0.2
Total Other Income	60.00	0.3	420.00	0.2
Net Income (Loss)	6,500.00	33.3	51,000.00	25.7

Figure 1.6   Sample Profit and Loss (P&L)/Income Statement with Year-to-Date (YTD) Comparison

BALANCE SHEET

Assets

    Assets

Cash on Hand (petty cash)	$ 50.00	
Cash in Bank	2,000.00	
Cash in Savings	10,000.00	
Total Assets		<u>$12,050.00</u>

    Fixed Assets

Equipment	10,000.00	
Furniture & Fixtures	1,000.00	
Office Equipment	4,000.00	
Computer & Printer	1,000.00	
Accumulated Depreciation	(4,000.00)	
A/D Equipment	(4,000.00)	
A/D Office Equipment	(1,000.00)	
A/D Office Equipment	(4,000.00)	
Total Fixed Assets		<u>$3,000.00</u>

Total Assets		$15,050.00

Liabilities

    Liabilities
    Long-Term Liabilities

Loan	20,000.00	
Total Long-Term Liabilities		$20,000.00

Total Liabilities		$20,000.00

Capital

Prop – Capital Account	(10,000.00)	
Prop – Drawing	(20,000.00)	
Prop – Deductible Draw	(3,000.00)	
Current Earnings	33,000.00	
Total Capital		($4950.00)

Total Liabilities and Capital		$15,050.00

Figure 1.7   Sample Balance Sheet for Start-up Sole Proprietorship

ed (i.e., those not yet collected), but indicates profitability of a department and percentage ratios of expenses to revenues.

A freestanding department will also be interested in a balance sheet report, which summarizes the business' assets, liabilities, and capital at a given time (Bangs, 1998a) See Figure 1.7 for a Sample Balance Sheet.

The P & L should be compared to the proposed budget for the first year to three years of the department's operation. Initially, determining whether targeted figures were appropriate will assist in future budgeting. Eventually, the P & L becomes a tool to guide the manager in program planning, financial analysis, and future projections. When analyzing a P&L report it is important to note that any losses are indicated on the report with parentheses or brackets around the figures.

The questions below can be raised to challenge the assumptions of the proposed budget and direct the planning of future budgets:

- Has the expected revenue been realized?
- Are expenses in line with projections?
- If discrepancies exist, why?
- What percentage of the revenue is spent on expenses?
- Can/should changes be made in the department to increase profitability?
- Are opportunities being lost due to lack of staff?
- Does waste in spending exist in any area?
- What percentage of total revenues is each line item (e.g., staff salaries and benefits constitute 80 percent of expenses)?
- Are there any expenses that should be reduced or added?

Additional financial analysis can include the comparison of monthly and year-to-date P & Ls from the previous year. Observe trends in revenues as well as expenses. Profitability is highly variable depending on market type and location but should be compared to itself for purpose of analysis.

Summary

Initializing an OT program or practice requires considerable motivation, leadership skills, planning, and justification for success to be realized. By understanding personal, professional, and political limitations, the program is more likely to avert unexpected setbacks. Solomon (1991) identifies some key factors in the success of a practice. They are location, cost effectiveness, superior or unique skills, marketing skills, and reputation for innovation. If these are achieved, the department manager is likely to have prepared adequately for a new program.

Always striving for the delivery of quality services should be the primary aspect of the mission. Placing consumer care as the focus of a therapy department is likely to assure confidence from referral sources.

Careful budgeting and staff management are among those tasks incumbent upon the OT manager. Keeping these issues at the forefront of planning, while holding a vision for future program expansion, will pave the way for a positive start to a developing program.

Case Study 1

An OT manager in a large hospital system has been asked to develop a satellite clinic specializing in early intervention and pediatrics. The present OT department, which supplies an in-patient and outpatient hospital setting with occupational therapy services, consists of five OTs, two OTAs, one full-time receptionist, and one part-time aide. Three OTs and one OTA are full-time employees. The remainders are half-time (20 hour per week) employees. The caseloads of four of the therapists indicate that they are only 40% productive at this time.

A $20,000.00 equipment budget has been allocated. Space has been designated but the amount of square footage is to be determined. The responsibilities of the manager include determining space requirements, ordering supplies and equipment, staffing, and establishing an annual budget.

Discussion Questions

1. Will the manager need to hire additional staff for this satellite clinic? How were these decisions reached?

2. Make a list of capital and operating expenses anticipated. Stay within the $20,000.00 budget allowed.

3. Describe the space required for this program. Include square footage needs and how it will be utilized.

4. How will the mission statement guide the manager in planning, decision-making, marketing, and the budgeting?

5. Develop a budget using a profit and loss statement (P&L). Include the expected revenues and expenses at start-up and after the first year of operation.

6. What vision do you expect the manager to have about future expansion of this satellite clinic?

Case Study 2

An industrial rehabilitation private practice has operated for 5 years with adequate profits and a flexible budget. Steady growth has been realized, but although finances are stable, referrals have plateaued over the last six months. An established hospital based program has opened a new on-site program following extensive training of one of their industrial rehabilitation staff. It has also increased its marketing in the area of on-site industrial rehabilitation programs. Referral sources report that new programs by the competitor are beneficial to patient progress. In addition, changes in legislation are being proposed which may reduce reimbursement for injured workers who have not yet returned to work.

Discussion Questions

1. What response should the OT manager take to the competitor's new program?

2. Is the plateauing of referrals a concern?

3. What should the OT manager do regarding possible legislative changes?

4. Write a SWOT (strength, weakness, opportunities, and threats) analysis for this program.

Case Study 3

An outpatient clinic has one full-time OT, one part-time OT (20 hours per week), one full-time OTA, and one part-time OTA (20 hours per week).

Discussion Questions

1. If a quarter-hour charged for occupational therapy is $40.00 and each therapist remains 60% productive for 45 weeks per year, what is the annual projected revenue for this department?

2. If annual salaries total $105,000.00 and total expenses for the year are $50,000.00, will this department experience a net profit in this example? What is the ratio of revenues to expenses?

3. Are any changes indicated?

CHAPTER 2

Program Growth, Expansion, and Community Practice Options

With time and creativity, an existing department may expand to include services into other areas of practice, additional locations, and/or a wider range of consumers. If expansion is to be successful, adequate staff must be available and employees' levels of expertise evaluated. Competence and quality in all areas must be assured.

Because legislative and reimbursement changes have and will continue to have an impact on the services provided by occupational therapists, nontraditional settings have emerged as options for the implementation of occupational therapy opportunities. To move into this broader frame of reference, the occupational therapist must be able to identify and market the strengths intrinsic to the profession.

At the conclusion of this chapter, the reader will be able to:

1. Identify community practice options for the occupational therapist.
2. Obtain information on federal, state, and local grant availability.
3. Develop a contract for providing OT services to agencies.
4. Determine appropriate expansion opportunities for existing programs.

Expanding Occupational Therapy Into Nontraditional Settings

Limitless opportunities exist for OTs in the face of change. Many nontraditional settings are emerging as areas of practice, often where OT was previously not utilized. Hospitals, nursing homes, schools, home health settings, and day treatment and outpatient settings are expected to continue to employ OTs. However, looking beyond these traditional practice areas will positively impact the profession and create employment opportunities where few existed in the past.

When researching possible community practice areas, Internet searches, telephone books, newspapers, agency brochures, and regional chambers of commerce can offer a wealth of information about community resources. Inquiries with community agency directors and staff can guide the occupational therapy program developer towards the needs of recipients. Thinking "outside the box" requires good understanding of the strengths of occupational therapy as a profession. The ability to market these strengths can lead to opportunities in settings that may have never considered utilizing the services of an occupational therapist. Vacant positions allocated for other professionals may be suited for the services of an occupational therapist, and if an agency does not recognize it, it is incumbent upon the OT to self-advocate! Good promotion and representation of what occupational therapy has to offer is necessary for this to be successful. Chapter 5, Marketing the OT Program or Clinic, describes marketing oneself and the profession of occupational therapy.

Nationally, occupational therapists have had to become creative in defining their roles in health care following the 1997 Balanced Budget Act. When many OTs were no longer employed in traditional settings, it was necessary to reevaluate the contribution and cost effectiveness of OT to the consumer.

The American Occupational Therapy Association (AOTA) describes occupational therapy as "a health and rehabilitation profession that helps people regain, develop, and build skills that are important for independent functioning, health, well-being, security, and happiness." From this definition it can be concluded that expanded visionary thinking will reveal many settings where these skills can be utilized.

Developing occupational therapy programs at the community level often requires being responsive to global changes in society and legislation. Keeping informed of governmental issues regarding health and social services will alert interested parties to federal and state issues. Grants or bills compatible to the services provided by occupational therapists can then be targeted.

By registering for Internet data links, ongoing resources about specific areas of interest can be received via e-mail, including notification about legislative bills passed, defeated, or in process, finances allocated, and/or amendments made.

Seeking Community Agency Contracts

Begin any interaction with nontraditional agency settings by becoming familiar with the facility's mission statement, its functions, and its reputation. Investigate the programs provided, their funding sources, and population served. Research staff positions and degrees held, if possible. Look at staff skills and backgrounds. Question present utilization of occupational therapy and the agency's understanding of the services occupational therapists can offer.

To begin program development in nontraditional settings, follow these steps:

1. Identify gaps in programming that occupational therapists may fill.

2. Contact the key individuals of the agency, e.g., program director, human resource manager, safety director, case manager, business owner and/or operator, board of directors.

3. Set up a meeting to discuss the purpose and intentions of the proposed services and to clarify questions found in research of facility.

4. Ask for a tour and/or orientation to the agency.

5. Explain the use of OT services in this setting.

6. Write a plan or proposal emphasizing the benefits the facility would receive by utilizing occupational therapy. Include the financial impact: how money can be saved, how added revenue can be produced, or how the budget can be accommodated. Illustrate time frames for implementation, resources required, and anticipated outcomes. See Figure 2.1 for an example of written program justification.

MEMO

TO:

DATE: March 12, 2001

SUBJECT: New Program Justification
Multi-Sensory Treatment Clinic

CC:

With a greater number of elementary and high school aged children requiring medication and/or suffering from Attention Deficit Disorder (ADD), and Attention Deficit Hyperactivity Disorder (ADHD), as well as all the varieties of autistic conditions prevalent today, it seems evident that an approach to helping these children learn in school would be a most valuable service to the community. The proposed program described below would meet the needs of this population by offering a program designed to address the multi-sensory needs of the child with the goal to prepare them for after school homework and daily living tasks. A tutoring service could also be implemented as well, following the treatment session. A more detailed description of the program is described below:

PROGRAM DESCRIPTION

A multi-sensory, sensory integration clinic for children and young adults who are challenged by dysfunctional sensory processing which interferes in their ability to complete school and/or work assignments. The 30-minute treatment session will be provided on a one-on-one basis. An individual program will be developed based on each participant's sensory profile. The stimulation or inhibition offered may include music, lights, textures, colors, visual, and auditory input, e.g., bubble and lava lamps, and color wheel. Comfortable lounging on a beanbag chair, hammock, or swing can further facilitate a calming atmosphere. A plastic ball pool is also available for appropriate individuals.

Following each session, the individual is required to work with their attendant, tutor, parent, or guardian for a minimum of 30 minutes to complete previously established work.

The outcome of the program will be determined by the goals(s) attainment over 3-month intervals. It is expected that an established project or assignment(s) will be completed during each quarter. Charges will be based on a 1-hour session, including one-half hour of one-on-one with a therapist, and the remainder supervised by the therapist. Charges will be _____ dollars per hour.

The program is expected to seek 5 patients per week initially, with growth potential to 10 within 6 months. Revenue for this project is identified as _____ dollars per month growing to _____ dollars per month, within 1 year. Although present net profits are projected as only _____ dollars per month, it is an opportunity to create a new market niche that is valuable to the community.

In addition, the space to be used has not been well utilized in the last 6 months.

Investment for start-up equipment and supplies is approximately _____ dollars. Ongoing supplies are minimal with primary expense being OT salaries.

Because there is an occupational therapist on staff with interest in the program and she presently notes there is time in her schedule, it is an opportune time to implement this program. The program would be implemented in an off-site clinic on Jones Street, which is in a convenient location to the schools.

FUNDING

The Health and Family Services Learning Resources Program as a supplement to private and non-government insurance policies will provide funding. A program would be available to students during pre-homework times of the day such as directly after the school day.

Figure 2.1   New Program Justification *(continues)*

MARKETING

Marketing these new services will be done through personal contact with potential referring sources. The program will be coordinated with Health and Human Services and the Lakeside School District. These parties have both been involved in the initial discussion stages of this program and are in full support of its inception. It is recommended that development of the program and implementation of it begin for the fall term of 2002-03, coordinated with the school calendar schedule.

Figure 2.1   New Program Justification (*continued*)

Provide marketing and educational materials to describe the benefits of OT to program directors, staff, referral sources, and decision makers.

Assist the agency in finding funding sources if necessary. Private insurance, entitlement programs, public assistance, government or private grant, and private donations may be accessed. Finally, if services are provided, be sure to monitor and document the outcomes/benefits of the occupational therapy services. If the contract or services are provided on a limited basis, make sure that occupational therapy's impact will continue in the future by training staff or family, providing resources, and leaving reports and recommendations. If possible, empower the program to function independently after occupational therapists are no longer present.

Grant Writing

As a whole, occupational therapists may need to be less dependent upon third party payers and look for other ways to implement the talents of the profession. Many can benefit by occupational therapy services when provided in other arenas not typically acknowledged. For example, federal grant funds allocated to families of special needs children may be spent on programs carried out by an occupational therapist.

Depending upon the type of grant available, colleges, hospitals, school districts, and non-profit and for-profit organizations may qualify for grant funding. State and federal dollars are allocated to general *and* specific categories. This money can be accessed through the grant application process. To be successful when applying for a grant, an organization must identify what sets it apart from other grant seekers. Demonstrating differing methods and approaches, expected outcomes, and how the program plans to meet the goals of the funding source may increase the success of the efforts, according to David Bauer (1995).

Grant Seeking

A grant can be approached in two ways: 1) An individual has a proposal idea and looks for a funder with a compatible vision for its implementation, e.g., a therapist develops a method/research model that is expected to significantly decrease health care costs, so the OT manager seeks out a grant focusing on health care cost reduction; 2) Prospective granters are researched with a general focus and the proposal is then defined accordingly, e.g., searches are completed using key words such as risk youth, underprivileged children, or special needs foster care. In both cases, the World Wide Web is useful to locate grant resources and availability.

Developing a Grant Proposal

An organized project is one that is documented from the initial stages through completion. A written proposal requires a strategic approach to its implementation. Bauer (1995) considers the following areas when justifying a grant proposal:

1. The program and solution
2. The result if left unaddressed
3. The present unmet need and vision for how it could be fulfilled
4. The urgency of spending funds on this proposal

Because documenting need is an important part of grant proposal, a needs assessment is recommended. Obtaining information from case studies, public forums, interviews of key players, data analysis, random surveys, and research of literature are recommended by Bauer (1995). A proposal is more likely to succeed if the funder believes there is a compelling need for the project, the project is supported by the organization's mission, and the proposed organization is well qualified to implement the plan. The reader is referred to Bauer (1995) for more detailed information on successful grant writing.

Types of Grants

The federal government granted 90 million dollars in 1999, foundations and corporations together awarded 21.6 billion dollars, according to Bauer (1995). It is important to comprehend the purpose of each grant, in order to narrow the focus of the market to be tapped. Among government grants, block, project or research, formula, contracts, and state government grants are options.

The block grant refers to a group of related programs that were combined as a "block" and dispersed directly to the states. Each state then establishes individual priorities and awards funds to projects accordingly.

Project or research grants are designed to attract specific projects of concern to the federal government. Some examples for occupational therapy may be reduction of Medicare expenditures, programs to decrease violence in children, increasing job skills for Welfare To Work program recipients, or fostering self-esteem in at-risk youth. These funds are allocated by Congress through authorized government programs and contain specific guidelines for implementation. Due to the ever-changing political climate, awareness of fund reallocation and shifts in focus of agenda is important.

Formula grants determine a set of criteria or formula to qualify for granting programs. Numbers of individuals, e.g., illiterate high school graduates, office workers with carpal tunnel syndrome, percentage of persons, and other census data fall into this category. These funds are focused on the areas of health, criminal justice, and employment. A defined problem or geographical region will increase eligibility for formula grants.

Contracts are slightly different from grants. Detailed government specifications and guidelines must be followed under a contract. The federal contracting agency must be confident the program will be completed with acceptable competency and at the lowest cost (Bauer, 1995).

State government grants are often federally allocated dollars which are passed to the grant seeker through individual states. Health and social welfare initiatives are often created by states, which distribute monies to address these needs accordingly.

Because federal block and formula grants are utilized, state government grants may be accessed more easily. Although states may impose their own restrictions, federal rules must be followed in project implementation.

Grant Searches

A number of resources are used for identifying federal and state grant availability. The Commerce Business Daily (CBD), a government contracting institute, provides products, publications, and services to its members about targeting, winning, and performing contracts. It publishes a list of available government contracts at www.cbd.com. These types of grants have been popularized by non-profit organizations, possibly due to large amounts of funds available. It is anticipated that the inexperienced contract bidder may have difficulty securing these funds, however, and should seek guidance from an experienced contract bidder.

Another of the available sites for identifying all aspects of government contracting is http://www.govsales.net. Members receive information and strategies to obtain some of the billions of dollars awarded annually for state, federal, and local contracts.

In addition, the reader is directed to http://www.fdncenter.org and http://www.access.gpo.gov/sudocs/aces/aces/40.html for federal grant register and foundation information.

See Figure 2.2 for a listing of federal research tools (Bauer, 1995).

Catalog of Federal Domestic Assistance—phone #202-512-1800; Fax 202-512-2250; online at www.gsa.gov/fdac/default.hgm.

Federal Assistance Programs Retrieval System (FAPRS)—phone #202-708-5126 or 1-800-669-8331.

Federal Register—phone #202-512-1800; Fax 202-512-2250; online at www.nara.gov/fedreg/.

U.S. Government—phone #202-512-1800; Fax 202-512-2250; online at www.access.gpo.gov/

Federal Directory—phone #202-333-8620.

Commerce Business Daily—phone #202-512-1800; Fax 202-512-2250; online at www.cbdnet.access.gpo.gov/.

Congressional Record—phone #202-512-1800; Fax 202-512-2250; online at www.access.gpo.gov/su/docs/aces/aces150.html.

Listing of Government Depository Libraries—phone #202-783-3238; online at www.access.gpo.gov/su_docs/libpro.html.

Federal Grant Circulars can be obtained from www.doleta.gov/regs/omb/index.htm or ordered from Superintendent of Documents Government Printing Office, Washington, DC 20402-9238; ph: 202-512-1800.

Figure 2.2. Federal Research Tools Worksheet (Bauer, 1995)

Catalog of Federal Domestic Assistance (CFDA). The CDFA lists 71,300 granting programs which can be accessed via hard copy or the Internet. Hard copy users must be familiar with the index. It contains:

- Agency Program Index—information on agencies administering programs. Must know the agency names to use this index.
- Applicant Eligibility Index—identifies qualifications for eligibility.
- Deadline Index—contains deadlines for dates of submission.
- Functional Index—20 broad categories and 176 subcategories such as education.
- Subject Index—the most commonly used, subjects list grants.

Clicking on the query catalog provides Internet access to CFDA. Questions to perform a search are found. Information provided includes:

- Program, number, and title
- Federal agency
- Authorization
- Objectives
- Types of assistance
- Uses and use restrictions
- Eligibility requirements
- Application and award process
- Assistance consideration
- Post-assistance requirements
- Financial information
- Program accomplishments
- Regulations, guidelines, literature
- Information contacts
- Related programs
- Examples of funded projects
- Criteria for selecting proposals

Federal Register. The Federal Register documents provide daily updates of government activities related to national archives and records administration. Hard copy, CD-ROM, and Internet access is possible for users.

The grant seeker can find published notices, and rules and regulations about a program of interest after the best government-funding program has been chosen using the CFDA.

The Office of Management and Budget (OMB). The OMB provides access to standards for financial dealings with government granting agencies. Regulations can specify allowable cost, indirect cost rates, and accounting requirements.

Home and Community Based Waiver Programs

Medicaid home and community-based service (HCBS) waivers allow states to develop alternatives to placing Medicaid-eligible individuals in institutions such as hospitals, nursing facilities, or intermediate care facilities for persons with mental retardation. This program acknowledges that these individuals may be cared for in less restrictive environments which allow and promote greater independence at no greater cost than an institutional setting.

States can develop Medicaid funded home and community based services by applying for waivers of certain federal requirements in section 1902 of the Social Security Act. Among alternative programs which may be provided are: case management, homemaker/home health aide services, personal care services, adult day health care, habilitation, and respite care.

The impacts these waiver programs have on OT are in the content of services provided. Medicare and Medicaid entitlement programs generally reimburse for occupational therapy services. Therefore OT is marketable to waiver programs as enhancements of their programs by utilizing the skills inherent to the profession.

To find the latest summary of approved home and community based services go to www.hcfa/gov/medicaid/hpgl.htm. This website contains descriptions, requirements, and processes for the program and demonstration waivers.

Obtaining Community Feedback for Program Expansion

Consumer advocacy is a powerful method of obtaining community interest in a new service. A consumer advisory committee can be formed to provide feedback, ideas, and strategies for eliciting community support and implementing program expansion.

For example, an OT manager interested in pursuing the establishment of an arthritis support group may elicit feedback from members of the community. A focus group could be created with individuals from a variety of professions, including one or two persons with arthritis. Several meetings could be conducted to determine the need, feasibility, and community support for this type of program.

When is Status Quo O.K.?

There are times in the evolution of an occupational therapy program that a productive and content staff wish to continue their present level of service without taking on new projects. Other times, personal and family situations may prevent participants from extending themselves additionally in their professions(s). Burnout is also an acceptable reason for withholding expansion of services. If in any of these examples the individual is unable to be effective in the development of *quality* programming, additional services should be avoided until issues are resolved. Also, if all services provided in a geographical area are adequate for the consumer, then additional services may be unnecessary.

Support and Financing for Expansion

A new business plan may be required, including a financial plan, if a financial institution will be needed to fund the expansion. (See Chapter 3 for details about writing financial and business plans). Also, to obtain top management and financial support for new endeavors in an institutional setting, government agency, or other facility, a program description and proposal is often necessary.

Justification proposals serve to detail in writing the primary factors driving the vision. An oral presentation may be required as well. If this is the case, visual aids are recommended such as slides, graphs, and financial projections.

A sample document justifying program expansion within a facility is found in Figure 2.1.

The components of a document used to elicit support for program expansion may include, but are not limited to:

- Services provided
- Mission statement
- Benefit of program to community
- Identification of population served
- Staff and equipment requirements (including costs)
- Expected and projected profitability
- Revenues and expenses
- Additional space needed
- Specific objectives and methods to meet them
- Analysis of competition
- Market plan (See Chapter 5).

Types of Program Options

For the visionary, forward thinker, there are nearly infinite opportunities for the occupational therapist. Traditional types of OT programs have changed and progressed over the years, usually due to regulations related to reimbursement of OT services. For example, there have been drastic reductions in OTs over the last two decades in the areas of:

- Inpatient hospital settings due to Diagnostic Related Groups (DRGs).
- Inpatient chronic mental health facilities secondary to deinstitutionalization.
- Long-term care programs following the adoption of the Balanced Budget Act (BBA) of 1997, and the prospective payment system (PPS).

Initially, most saw these regulation changes as having a negative impact on the OT profession, which is often realized by the OT consumer! However, it is helpful to remember the old saying, "With every cloud there is a silver lining." For example, because of these changes, new opportunities presented themselves for the occupational therapist, including:

- Home health programs and sub-acute rehabilitation settings replaced long inpatient hospital stays.
- Day treatment centers, group homes, sheltered work, and community reentry programs were expanded in response to deinstitutionalization.
- Cost containment and functional outcomes were strengthened as a necessity to survive PPS, community practice options were created, and wellness programs justified.

If a therapist is flexible and a forward thinker, he or she can react and predict new avenues to pursue in the health care market, most always creating a benefit for the OT consumer where their needs were not being met. Presently, the following scenarios exist for occupational therapy services in the community.

Outpatient Clinics

Many types of clinics offer OT services to the consumer. They may include:

- Pediatrics

- Industrial rehabilitation
- General OT/rehabilitation services
- Hand therapy
- Wellness programs, stress management, biofeedback
- Sports injuries

School Systems

Contracts with individual school districts or the governing agencies controlling therapists in the districts fill the need for OT services in the educational environment. See Figure 2.3 for a sample contract with a school district.

On-site Industrial Rehabilitation and Wellness Programs

To comply with Occupational Safety & Health Administration (OSHA) ergonomic standards, many industries and businesses are becoming more open to offering:

- Prevention programs for back and neck injuries
- Carpal tunnel and cumulative trauma prevention classes
- Worksite ergonomics
- Stress reduction programs
- Onsite therapy services
- Office ergonomics

Managers and entrepreneurs interested in providing services to business and industry must become familiar with the OSHA proposed ergonomic standards, which can be downloaded from their web site www.osha.gov (O'Connor, 2000).

Contracts with Hospitals, Home Health Agencies, and Nursing Homes

Some agencies prefer to contract for rehabilitation services, especially if their need is small or positions are hard to fill. Providing vacation, on-call, and fill-in services is an excellent way to initiate a private practice.

Sheltered Workshops

The expertise of an occupational therapist is a valuable tool in the supervised work setting. Frequently, OTs are often underutilized in this environment. Services are appropriate for:

- Ergonomics
- Work simplification/adaptation
- Perceptual motor intervention
- Cognitive skills training
- Independent living services: meal preparation, homemaking, community integration, self-help, transportation
- Psychosocial interactions: peer interaction, work behaviors

AGREEMENT BETWEEN _____
AND _____

_____ and _____ mutually agree to the conditions listed below:

1. _____ will provide the following services to the School District of _____:

   a. Provide occupational therapy as described in each Individualized Educational Plan for students on the assigned caseload. The services will be provided in the school at which student is enrolled.

   b. Participate in the development of IEPs for students on the assigned caseload assuring that the occupational therapy services depicted on the IEPs will be implemented accurately as identified in the established IEP.

   c. Participate in placement committee meetings for students on the assigned caseload.

   d. Complete occupational therapy reevaluations and participate in the three year reevaluation meetings for students on the assigned caseload.

   e. Complete occupational therapy initial evaluations and participate in evaluation team meetings for students assigned.

   f. Request an IEP meeting and assist the IEP committee in revising a student's IEP when occupational therapy services are no longer recommended for a student.

   g. Participate in Section 504 Identification/Accommodation meetings when assigned by School Psychologist.

   h. Serve as a consultant to _____ School District on occupational therapy and assistive technology issues as well as other special education issues.

   I. Comply with all requirements and timelines related to the provision of occupational therapy in _____ Administrative Code Chapter _____, _____ School District policy.

2. _____ will maintain the appropriate documentation for students on the assigned caseload for purposes of third party reimbursement.

3. The occupational therapist designated to provide the services specified in the agreement is approved by the _____ School District. He/she will have a current _____ Department of Regulation and Licensing Occupational Therapist/Occupational Therapist Assistant certification.

4. _____ will submit a schedule to the Special Education Director identifying when services will be provided for each student on the caseload.

5. _____ will submit a log of hours to _____ on a bi-monthly basis, specifying the number of hours and the type of service provided.

6. _____ School District will pay _____ per above invoice at a rate of $_____ per hour for services rendered.

7. The agreement is effective from July 1, _____ through June 30, _____. Renewal of contract will be based on mutual agreement of both parties.

8. _____ may use the services of an occupational therapy assistant (OTA) to provide direct services to students if, a.) in _____ professional judgment, the quality of occupational therapy will not be diminished, b.) the assistant holds the appropriate _____ Department of Public Instruction license, and c.) the specific individual providing the therapy is agreed to by the _____ School District. All services provided by an Occupational Therapist for consultation and supervision of OTA will also be approved by _____ at the _____School District.

Figure 2.3   Sample Contract for OT Services with School District *(continues)*

9. The _____ School District will provide space and supplies necessary for completion of occupational therapy services as required to meet the goals stated in the IEP for each student.

10. The _____ School District will pay travel time in the amount of $_____ per hour for each visit to render OT services, participate in IEP, E-team meetings, supervise OTA, and for evaluations performed by the occupational therapist.

11. Both parties will make significant effort to coordinate IEP meetings during regular scheduled visits to _____ School District by the occupational therapist. The occupational therapist will make every effort to attend all meetings, however if scheduling conflict occurs, a conference call and/or a prior meeting with parent(s)/OTR, including documentation, will be completed.

12. _____ will schedule all therapy and evaluation times with individual classroom teacher taking into consideration the best interest of the student's educational experience.

13. _____. will provide OT services up to ____ hours per week __% FTE unless requested by school district.

_____

School District Representative/Date

_____

Facility Representative/Date

Figure 2.3   Sample Contract for OT Services with School District *(continued)*

Community Service Agencies

Government funded programs often need the assistance of an occupational therapist but frequently are unsure of what OT provides. Educating local social service agencies can open doors for community services in the areas of:

- In-home therapy
- Birth-to-three intervention
- Group home programs
- Assisted living services

Wellness Programs

Private pay situations exist in some locations. Aquatic therapy, movement therapy, therapeutic touch, relaxation, therapeutic exercise are all areas in which the occupational therapist may provide services to the community. Frequently, however, these programs may not be reimbursable and, therefore, would most often be feasible in geographical locations where private pay customers exist.

Insurance Companies and Worker's Compensation Carriers

Case management has emerged as a legitimate means of cost containment. OTs have the background and skills to fill the role of case manager, providing this service to the insurance company, which saves health care costs while offering a liaison between the insurance carrier and the consumer.

Well Elderly Programming

Fall prevention services, senior fitness, aquatic therapy, and in-home independent living strategies are all examples of appropriate avenues for the OT to pursue.

In-home Care for the Disabled

There is a major focus nationally for supportive home care for individuals with disabilities in lieu of nursing facilities or other institutions. Current legislation drafted by American Disabled for Attendant Programs Today (ADAPT) in 1999, the Medicaid Community Attendant Services and Supports Act (MiCASSA) will give the disabled population, including the elderly, the rights to community, in-home care. At the time this information was written, MiCASSA was not approved, and was in the process of being refined. In addition, the Olmstead decision is a Supreme Court decision stating that services for the disabled must be offered in the community. Occupational therapists can market themselves as a service that not only restores maximal functional ability in this population but as a discipline able to determine supportive care needs for in-home care. Visit www.adapt.org/casa for updated information on this bill.

Nontraditional Placements

One's imagination may be among the only limiting factors in the future of occupational therapists. The skills possessed by the OT are invaluable in numerous nonmedical arenas for training, consultation, cost reduction, supervision, and direct care, when the outcome is to increase function and independence in the recipient. See Figure 2.4 for a listing of options for community practice programs. Services can be delivered to individuals, groups, families, and teams in the private and public sector. Government contracts and grants provide possibilities to the OT willing to pursue them.

Impacting Legislation: Being an Advocate for Occupational Therapy

It will behoove the OT manager and all OTs and OTAs to become familiar with their legislative representatives. Although for many this appears a daunting task, it is actually the job of the representative to become familiar with the views of his or her constituents. Therefore, they will welcome contact from constituents and are generally eager to meet with them. Keeping this in mind should help to reduce the "fear factor" in approaching government officials.

There are some things to keep in mind when contacting those holding government offices:

- They are "in session" at the state capitol during generally predictable times of the year and alternate their time in their home region.
- Initial contact is made with an aide in the legislator's office, where the legislator's schedule can be determined and appointments set up.
- Offer to meet in their office, but be patient. The may have only brief periods of time, may get called out of the meeting, or may cancel at the last minute. Always be courteous and congenial. If necessary, walk along beside the legislator and plead your case efficiently while they are heading to their next commitment.

Adoption agencies and foster care agencies

Child care centers

Churches

Community based residential care facilities (CBRFs)

Community health and wellness centers

Computer sales offices and businesses

Free health clinics

Group home and independent living centers

Immigration agencies

Industrial and manufacturing facilities

Job training and coaching agencies

Native American communities

Playground architectural companies

Programs and/or housing for individuals with HIV, AIDS

Recreation programs, urban or rural

Renovation, architect, and construction companies

Senior centers and day programs

Sheltered workshop settings

Shelters for the homeless and battered women

Welfare to work programs

Youth centers

Vocational rehabilitation programs

Figure 2.4 Community Practice Options .

- Meeting with them out of their office requires flexibility on the therapist's part, but legislators are usually willing to accommodate a luncheon, state association dinner, awards presentation, or small social gatherings with family, friends, and neighbors.

- Be prepared for the meeting. Be familiar with the issue(s) being presented and advocate for the benefits of OT services to the consumer. Give real life examples. Legislators are interested in what affects their constituents.

- Be willing to meet with the aide who works with the legislator. They are responsible for relaying all information back to the legislator, so the information will not be overlooked.

- Bring written material to leave with them. Written material should be concise, usually one sheet of paper that describes the issue briefly.

- Ask how they stand on the issue presented. Get a feel of how they may vote if the concern is a proposed bill or amendment.

- Never alienate an official by arguing or becoming angry if an agreement is not reached. Accept a negative response graciously, remembering that this individual may be needed for other issues in the future. Do not be intimidated by a difference of opinion.

- Always follow up the meeting with a thank you letter.

- The people elect them and the legislators job is to understand the issues of their constituents. Many are interested in reelection, and are very appreciative of those interested in volunteering on campaigns or donating funds.

There are many other ways to impact the legislature to get specific proposals and bills on the "floor." AOTA has a very easy method on their website for members. The government relations area addresses current issues of importance to OTs. On the website the therapist can find a pre-drafted letter regarding the issue, with space available for additional comments, which will be linked to the individual's congressional representatives by entering the demographic information requested. The OT wishing to submit this letter can do so without even knowing their representative, the address, phone number, or email address!

Other methods of impacting legislation are to call the representative's office, send a letter, or email directly. To obtain information about the current representatives for a specific geographical area, contact the state OT office in the appropriate geographical location.

A telephone tree may also be utilized to rally support from multiple parties. Obtaining interest from other special interest groups can be helpful in implementing mass support as well. Using the press to bring attention to an issue via an editorial or article in a newspaper may spark interest in critical issues from many constituents and get the attention of the representative.

Summary

Development of *quality* programming and services should always be the priority when program expansion is considered.

Successful program expansion requires significant thought, planning, and finances. It is time consuming and if performed with little planning and effort, the results can be less effective.

Creating and expanding opportunities for OT services independent of traditional settings will maximize benefits to the community. This is made possible by using visionary leadership and management, researching funding options, and targeting gaps in community services.

Case Study 1

A department manager is faced with an opportunity to create a market niche in the area of home health care. The manager presently supervises a program with three staff: two OTs and one OTA (all full-time). Productivity is 100% for two staff and 50% for the third position. The manager worries that it may not be possible to operate a new program with a half-time position, especially due to the travel involved. On the other hand, hiring another staff person could be risky.

The idea of participating in the home health care arena began when frequent telephone calls were noted at the clinic inquiring about OT services in the home. The individuals reported inability to obtain timely service and were placed on a waiting list for up to two weeks.

Discussion Questions

1. What steps should the manager take to determine feasibility of a market share in home health care?
2. Should a fourth staff person be hired? If so, why and when? If not, why not?
3. Should the position be part-time or full-time?
4. What equipment and supplies would be necessary for the new program?

Case Study 2

A bill is proposed in the legislature that would eliminate OT services from coverage in the schools under Public Law.

Discussion Questions

1. How should this issue be addressed?
2. Write a letter to your representatives expressing your views.
3. Substantiate your views in a newspaper editorial.
4. What other methods can be used to address this critical issue?

Case Study 3

An OT manager has developed a program for promoting and increasing self-esteem in children from families of alcoholic or chemically dependent parents.

Discussion Questions

1. Identify grant funds available for this type of program.
2. Who qualifies for the funding?
3. How much money is available?
4. How could this program be implemented in the community?

Discussion Topic #1

Choose from one of the following three scenarios and answer the questions below.

- Homeless shelter
- Independent living center for the chronic mentally ill

- Sheltered workshop

1. What services do you envision for this program?

2. What funds would be available for reimbursement?

3. Who would you contact with to arrange these services?

4. Call a community program listed on Figure 2.4 to determine the presence of occupational therapy services and what type of reimbursement is accessed for payment of OT.

CHAPTER 3

The Development of a Private Practice

Every small business begins with an idea of a service or product to be offered. A vision about a potential OT market requires substantiation of need before making the dream a reality. Becoming a private practitioner requires strong persistence, commitment, and flexibility. Because a financial obligation is assumed, the ability to accept a risk is also a quality the entrepreneur must possess.

At the conclusion of this chapter, the reader will be able to:

1. Perform market research to determine feasibility of a new practice.
2. Write a business plan and loan proposal.
3. Understand the differences between each business entity and choose the appropriate one for the proposed practice.
4. Establish the type and space requirements of a practice.
5. Set up a business office management system.

Market Research

Before a decision to start a practice is confirmed, one must establish a need for the type of service proposed. The questions below will offer a place to start when determining need in a market. There are two primary areas to investigate when considering an OT private practice. They are geographical location and level of competition.

1. Geographical location

   What is the population base requiring OT?

   How well are consumers' needs presently being met?

   What is the potential for referral sources in the area?

   What is the industrial base? In other words, what businesses and manufacturing facilities are operating there?

2. Level of competition

   Who is the competition?

   What are the strengths and weakness of the competition?

   What is the comparison to the competition? How would this new business differ from others who are providing a similar service?

Market research helps to answer the above questions. It can be performed by a professional consultant trained in methods of obtaining information about market trends and product need. But if a tight budget exists, marketing students interested in a research project may suffice. Some OT managers choose to complete market assessments independently.

If the information is to be gathered by the potential business owner, the process should not be taken lightly. A private practice begun without appropriate research may save time and money initially, but could be lacking valuable information to begin a new program. The steps listed below can guide the entrepreneur to greater understanding of the market for OT services in a specified geographical location.

Obtain Demographic Data

Demographic data can be obtained by contacting the local chamber of commerce, libraries, Internet searches, service clubs, government agencies, economic development agencies, Small Business administration programs, departments of commerce, trade publications, local trade associations, and telephone books.

The following items should be considered when searching for the market data.

- Population trends (e.g., retirement communities, young family developments, active adults, sports teams)
- Age of individuals (e.g., number and types of schools, nursing homes, senior centers, percentage of working age)
- Types of businesses (e.g., blue collar, professional, medical, educational)
- Growth or decline of business/industry (e.g., recent changes, presence of new or closing businesses, type of insurance provided)
- Number of employees in each business (e.g., lay-offs, types of injuries)
- Types of health care services (e.g., specialty services, amount of travel required to obtain)
- Providers of rehabilitation services (e.g., what therapy programs exist?)

Identify the "Consumer"

There are many consumers in the world of OT. Identify each one as a separate entity with different needs. The patient, resident, client, or student is the most obvious. Business owners and industry safety directors, physicians, other health care professionals, case managers, teachers and administrators, and government payer sources should not be overlooked as consumers as well. By confirming that each of these individuals plays a part as a consumer in the OT environment, the interaction with them will change. Each of their needs should be addressed differently and care should be taken to assure their satisfaction. For example, the business owner may need an ADA assessment; the safety director may need a work station consult, etc.

When defining the consumer, consider:

- Are the consumer's OT needs being met?
- What does the consumer want from OT?
- What is the potential to provide what the consumer is lacking?
- How does the consumer perceive the service to be provided?

- How large is the perceived consumer base?
- What is the type of reimbursement (if appropriate) of this consumer base?
- When do consumers use the service?
- What is the potential for repeat consumers?

Health Care Reimbursement

Determine primary types of health care reimbursement available. Contact large employers in the area to discern what health insurance carriers are used. The payer mix is important to the amount of reimbursement that can be expected. For example, if 50 percent of the population uses entitlement programs or is uninsured, the amount of actual payment for therapy services will be affected.

Make Initial Contact with Insurance Carriers

Begin the credentialing process to become part of preferred provider organizations (PPOs) and health maintenance organizations (HMOs), Medicare, Medical Assistance, Blue Cross/Blue Shield (BCBS), and other private insurance carriers in the geographical area where service will be performed. Applications must be requested and completed separately for each carrier. A provider number is given for each therapist if provider is approved. Group numbers are required by some payers for multi-provider facilities, and require a separate *group* application. Medicare requires use of a separate provider number for private practitioners when billing for durable medical equipment (DME). See Chapter 7, Reimbursement.

Determine Rates of Reimbursement for Current Procedural Terminology (CPT) Codes.

CPT coding is a national system using numbers to identify the procedure implemented. Reimbursement rates vary throughout the country, therefore, comparisons will be helpful when establishing fees for service. There are large discrepancies between managed care organizations, traditional insurance carriers, government agencies, and entitlement programs (Medicare and Medicaid) regarding rates of reimbursement. It must be noted here that government insurance programs, such as Medicare and Medicaid, and their recipients cannot be charged differently than other third party payers.

Complete Analysis of Current Rehabilitation and OT Services Offered

Make a list of present providers, facilities, and each service specialty. Document locations where these services are provided. Follow this with a list of perceived program inadequacies and/or groups of individuals being underserved.

Next, examine the compatibility of the proposed practice with the present market "gaps." This assessment of the market can function to form the direction of service delivery for the new practice.

Define the Competition

Although there can be overlap in services provided, a difference or uniqueness should be found in any new program offered. Look for the things that will set the new business apart from its competitors.

List the five closest competitors. Fine-tune the analysis to include five indirect or potential competitors. Find out:

- What services are provided
- What their charges are
- Who refers to them
- What is their financial stability
- How satisfied are previous patients with the service they received
- How satisfied are agencies with services received through contract

Compare proposed services with the competition in the areas of:

- Quality of service (including customer service and quality of outcomes)
- Cost of service
- Ease in access
- Location
- Financial stability
- Advertising
- Community perception
- Experience
- Mission
- Reputation

Information can be gathered in many ways. Printed materials such as brochures, annual reports, special fee literature, health fairs, libraries, chambers of commerce, and local service directories can provide valuable information.

Other methods of information retrieval are:

- Ask other OTs or rehabilitation staff what is known about the services and practices of the competition.
- Ask previous employees information about the services provided at a specific facility.
- Ask patients or former patients about the quality of therapy they received at a specific facility.
- Conduct a survey of the general public through direct mailing and/or telephone calls.
- Call the competitors and ask direct questions.
- Hold a focus group through public information.
- Be a "mystery shopper" by calling other providers to inquire as if you were a potential patient.

Identify Competitive Objectives (Bangs, 1998b)

- What is the competitive position of a program and how can it be improved? In other words, does the other program remain visible in the community through advertising, etc?

- What strengths of the proposed service can be targeted for purposes of marketing? For example, the presence of a specialty service, accessibility, evening or extended hours.

- Do the competitors have weaknesses that could be used to strengthen the new market? The competing program may lack evening hours or have minimal parking.

- How can the program learn from competitor's strengths? Good outcomes and strong referral sources to the competitor for some types of therapy, when coupled with a limited number of patients for that service, may indicate lack of future market need. If the competing service has a "corner on the market," it may be wise to avoid program development in this area of practice.

Identify and Contact Potential Referral Sources

Ask to meet with each individual to discuss some pertinent issues related to a new OT practice. Be persistent, it may take several calls or visits to get five to fifteen minutes of another individual's time (especially physicians). The American Occupational Therapy Association has identified a list of questions to ask potential referral sources (Crispen and Hertfelder, 1990):

A. Do your patients have OT needs that are not being met? If so, what are these needs?

B. Approximately how many patients do you refer and for what types of OT services in a year's time?

C. If you refer your patients for OT services, where do you refer them? Why?

D. What areas of OT service needs do you see as increasing?

E. What areas of OT service needs do you see as decreasing?

F. Are you totally satisfied with the current level of OT services your patients are receiving? If not, what could be done to improve these services?

G. Is there any way I can meet your office's OT needs in a way that would make it easier for you to obtain these services?

H. Do you currently receive the reports you need during and after the time OT services are provided to your patients?

I. On a scale of 1–10, how would you rate the services of _____?

J. What would it take to get you to switch some of your referrals to this proposed practice?

K. If a new practice is opened, will you agree to send three patients during the first six months to assure quality service?

Analyze the Market Research

By evaluating the findings of the market research, it should be clear what OT services are being provided. Existing needs in a geographical location for OT programs, satisfaction of referral sources with present programs, and their willingness to refer elsewhere should also be apparent. The strengths and weakness of existing departments should become evident after this process.

From this information, identify gaps in service, as well as the ability of a new practice to meet those service needs. If the new program being proposed is a duplication of another service offered, what would draw a customer or referral source to choose the new practice over the existing one?

Some reasons for consumer choice or change may include:

- Specialty versus general service offered
- Professional reputation, level of experience
- Convenience
- Personalized service
- Previous knowledge of therapist(s)
- Persistent marketing approach with strong education to community and referral sources
- Recommendation by physician
- Word of mouth

After completion and analysis of the market assessment, the type of practice, consumers, and specific services are defined. If not already completed, developing a mission statement (discussed in Chapter 1) including geographical area(s) served is the next step. Setting a price structure for procedures is a prerequisite to writing and outlining preliminary expenses and revenues.

Next, strategic planning is used as a method of clarifying the obstacles and understanding the steps for a successful business. Performing the strengths, weaknesses, opportunities, and threats (or SWOT) analysis, discussed in Chapter 1, is part of this process.

Defining the scope of practice, along with developing the mission and engaging in strategic planning, is the catalyst to writing a business plan for a new business. All OT practices should be established based upon the AOTA's "Standards of Practice" (Found in Appendix 1.2), which create a foundation for programs and will guide the manager during the planning and development stage.

Taking the Risk

Every individual has a different comfort level for taking risks. It cannot be overlooked that a business owner must be willing to tolerate a level of risk greater than that of an employee. To reduce the chance of catastrophic results due to potential risks, there are some steps to take:

- Identify the risks: injury to employee or consumers, harm or alleged harm to consumer, disabling condition to business owner or employees preventing ability to perform duties of the job, theft, fire, damage to property, decline in business, financial strain or loss.
- Purchase insurance: worker's compensation (required by law for all employees), unemployment compensation (required contribution by law), liability insurance (minimum of $2,000,000 to $4,000,000), umbrella policy ($1,000,000).
- Plan ahead: have a minimum of $5,000 to $10,000 available in a reserve account for unexpected incidents. Put this into the financial plan of the loan proposal.
- Do not take on too much too soon: be patient, build on services, gradually take on other expenses. Do not do *everything* initially.

Following good business practices and remaining ethical in all practices will allow the entrepreneur a good credit rating when looking for financing.

The Business Plan and Loan Proposal

The business plan is a written extension of the thoughts, ideas, and plans for a new business. It functions to define and direct a practice when starting out, expanding, obtaining financing, and/or making decisions. The completed plan is a tool for effective business management.

When seeking outside financing for the start-up of a private practice, a loan proposal is required. This is basically a business plan with more detailed financial information included for the benefit of the lender. The elements of a business plan and loan proposal are listed in order of presentation, with descriptions of each to follow (Bangs, Jr. 1998a; Pinson & Jinnett, 1996; Covello & Hazelgren, 1995; Crispen & Hertfelder, 1990.)

Elements of a Business Plan

1. Cover sheet
2. Table of contents
3. Executive summary
   a. Mission statement
   b. Plan purpose
4. Company summary
5. Service description
6. Customer description
7. Marketing
8. Management summary
9. Financial plan

Optional supporting documents may include:

> Personal resumes
> Personal balance sheets
> Credit reports
> Letters of reference
> Letters of intent
> Copies of leases
> Pertinent legal documents
> Contracts

A sample business plan is found in Appendix A-3.1. Descriptions of the primary contents of a business plan are outlined below.

Cover Sheet. There are differing opinions about the content of the cover sheet. It should always contain:

- Business name, address, and telephone number
- Owner(s) of business
- Date submitted

Additional information may include:

- Logo, if available
- Financial institutions applied to (if preparing a financial plan, use a separate cover sheet for each bank or source submitted to)
- Name of preparer

Executive Summary or Statement of Purpose (SOP). The first page of the document is to state the objectives, mission statement, and purpose of the plan. For example, "MVRC will be guided and operated by this plan for its initial and future decisions."

If a financial plan is required, also include in the SOP answers to the following questions (Bangs Jr., 1998a, 7):

1. Who is asking for money?
2. What is the business structure (e.g., sole proprietorship, partnership, corporation, limited liability corporation, or subchapter S corporation)?
3. How much money is needed?
4. How will the funds benefit the business?
5. Why does this loan or investment make business sense?
6. How will the funds be repaid?

Keep the SOP business-like and brief, usually no longer than one-half page.

Table of Contents (TOC). The TOC is not required but provides the reader a format for easy information retrieval. It falls at the beginning of the document and can be divided into three major categories:

1. The organization of the business
   a. Description of business
   b. Type of service
   c. Market share
   d. Location of office
   e. Competition outlook
   f. Staff considerations
   g. Marketing plan
2. Financial information
   a. Funding sources and application
   b. Balance sheet
   c. Fees for service
   d. Income projections: at one month, one year, and three years, (Figure 3.1)
   e. Profit and loss statement (Figure 1.6)
3. Additional optional documents.
   a. References
   b. Resumes
   c. Supporting information

Company Summary. The organization plan of the business contains details about critical information important to the reader and/or financial institution, including:

1. Description of business owner(s) including name, credentials, special training, skills, and experience.
2. Name of practice. Documentation about why the name was chosen is appropriate here. This is a brief statement to provide the reader some insight about the image to be projected.
3. Location of office. Where will the services be provided? If this is different than office location, where and how will the business management be conducted?

3-YEAR PROJECTIONS
PROFIT AND LOSS

	2000	2001	2002	2003
Sales	100,000	150,000	180,000	200,000
Minus cost of goods sold	5,000	7,000	10,000	10,000
Gross profit	95,000	143,000	170,000	190,000
Operating expenses				
Accounting and legal	2000	2500	2500	2700
Advertising	5000	3000	3000	3000
Bad debt	3000	3000	5000	3200
Dues & Subscriptions	500	600	600	800
Education	500	1000	1500	2000
Insurance	500	500	500	600
Interest-Loan	5000	6000	6000	6000
Rent	6000	6500	6750	7000
Salaries	70,000	90,000	100,000	100,000
Supplies	6000	7500	9000	10,000
Telephone	2500	2400	2500	2500
Travel & entertainment	1000	2000	2500	3000
Utilities	1200	1200	1200	1300
Total operating expense	103,200	126,200	141,050	162,100
Net income	-8,200	16,800	28,950	47,900

Figure 3.1. Income Projections; 3-year Profit and Loss

Service Description. This is a description of the services offered. Information about the following is found in this section, including:

> When will the business open?
>
> What are the types and ages of the population served?
>
> When will the services be provided throughout the week?
>
> What type of reimbursement is expected?
>
> What future plans are there for the business?

Customer Description

> Who are the primary sources of referral?
>
> Why will they refer or suggest the services of this new venture?
>
> How large is the suggested referral base and what is its potential for growth?
>
> What is the level of confidence in receipt of referrals?

Marketing

> Where are the gaps in this service?
>
> Why is it believed that this market is underserved?
>
> How can this business fill the gap?

What are the trends in this market?

Who are the primary competitors?

How does the proposed service compare and excel at providing it?

Why would a customer choose the proposed practice over the competition?

How is the new practice going to be introduced and marketed to the community?

What methods will be used to advertise and seek referrals?

What long-term marketing strategies will be considered?

Management and Staffing Requirements

What types and numbers of employees will be required to run the business?

What will the organizational structure be?

Financial Plan. This section can be brief if not applying for financial assistance from a bank or other lending agency. It should always include:

- Sources of financing
- Beginning balance sheet
- Annual projected income with justifications regarding trends in market and expectations for growth

Other information to include for thoroughness and when applying for a loan is (Pinson and Jinnett, 1996):

1. Summary of financial need.

   This section expresses why funds are requested, how much money is needed, and how the funds will serve to increase profits. Make sure the money borrowed with interest will work to strengthen revenues generated. Because at least six months worth of expenses may be required prior to a steady cash flow, this should be considered when requesting initial funds.

2. Table of Start-up Expenses (Figure 3.2).

   This is a description of how the funds will be used. Start-up costs, items purchased, capital and operating supplies, list of suppliers, price of items, marketing costs, salary costs, and consulting fees may be offered.

   A cash flow statement or budget is supplied in Figure 3.3. This section describes the finances of the business in a budget format. In preparation, the following data may be included:

   - Revenue projections (See Chapter 1)
   - Variable expenses—patient equipment, office supplies, marketing costs, bad debt, some utilities, and some wages.
   - Fixed expenses—salaries, some wages, lease, rent, loan, loan payments, some utilities.

3. Projected income statement

   This may be referred to as the profit or loss statement (P & L). It complements the balance sheet or cash flow statement. The balance sheet displays the business financial picture at a point in time. The P & L offers a look at a business's finances over a period of time, e.g., 3 years.

These documents are called proforma or projected financial documents. They are compilation of what the financial picture of a practice is *expected* to

Start-up Expenses	
Brochures	$500
Insurance	$500
Legal	$1,000
Office Supplies/Equipment	$2,000
Rent/Damage Deposit	$1,400
Printed Materials	$500
Total Start-up Expenses	$5,900
Start-up Assets Needed	
Cash Requirements	$5,000
Equipment	$5,000
Office Furniture	$2,000
Total Assets Needed	$12,000
Total Cash Needed for Start-up	$17,650
Investment:	
Jane Doe	$5,000
Short-Term Loans/Bank	$15,000
Total Financing	$20,000
Gains/Loss at Start-up	$2,350

Figure 3.2. Table of Start-up Expenses

Expected Gross Revenues	$75,000
Projected Expenses	
Accounting and legal	$2,000
Advertising	$2,400
Bad debt	$1,900
Dues & subscriptions	$500
Insurance	$700
Loan	$6,000
Rent	$5,000
Salaries	$40,000
Supplies	$5,000
Telephone	$1,500
Travel & entertainment	$1,500
Continuing Education	$1,000
Total Operating Expenses	$67,500
Projected Net Revenues	$7,500

Figure 3.3. Sample Annual Cash Flow Statement (Budget)

look like in the future. These figures are calculated on assumptions about case-loads, revenue received, market growth, economy, and trends.

"Income projections are forecasting and budgeting tools" (Bangs, Jr. 1998a). They supply the reader information about projected revenue and expenses. One, three, and five year P & Ls are standard. The first year should include monthly figures. Notes about trends and variations are helpful for future planning.

When projecting revenues, it is prudent to remember that increased revenue does not necessarily mean increased profit. Often, expenses increase with greater numbers on the caseload, for supplies, wages, etc. Therefore, the ratio between revenues received and expenses incurred will affect the analysis of the profit margin; or the profit realized *after* expenses.

In addition, an increase in *caseload* does not guarantee an increase in *revenues;* actual reimbursement rates vary with the payer. Monitoring the ratio of units produced (fees billed) and *actual* reimbursement will provide the practice with valuable financial information about effectiveness of fees collected.

Of note here is that managers often need to reflect upon financial information from a retrospective standpoint once programs are operating. By reviewing the budget in terms of what has already occurred, the manager can adjust expenses accordingly.

Although projected figures are not always targeted perfectly, experience and history will increase accuracy. If a category or section is grossly misread, making an adjustment for the future will extend the effectiveness of the document. See Figure 1.6 in Chapter 1 for sample income statement with one year and year-to-date (YTD) comparisons. These comparisons are valuable to future planning and are among the types of retrospective figures many managers rely on.

Supporting Documents (optional). Any information that will reinforce the documents provided in the business plan is relevant. Some suggestions for a start-up practice include:

1. Resume (see Chapter 1)—(must be provided)
2. Letters of reference—physicians, colleagues, previous business contacts, etc.
3. Letters of intent to refer by above sources
4. Lease agreements
5. Census/demographic information relevant to market share
6. Credit reports
7. Floor plans of proposed space (if building or remodeling)

Financing

There are a number of options available when borrowing money to set up a practice. The most common methods are as follows.

Term Loans

When issued, term loans must be repaid in a specified period of time (e.g., 5 years). Monthly payment plans are designed to include interest, usually based on a percentage above prime rate.

Line of Credit

A line of credit is issued as a specific amount of money for future purchases or expenses, and is utilized by the borrower, as the funds are needed. The line may stay "open" for a period of time, i.e., until the amount of money is used. During that time, only a monthly interest payment, paid only on the amount borrowed to that date, is required.

Receivable Financing

If a business is established, it can borrow funds against a percentage of the outstanding accounts receivable. New businesses usually do not qualify for this type of loan.

Small Business Loans

There are a variety of ways to qualify for a United States Small Business Administration (SBA) loan. Being denied a bank loan, qualifying for woman or minority status, or starting a business in certain locations may help a new business to obtain funds or guarantee a loan by the SBA. Typically the bank administrates the loan and the SBA insures against default. Contact the Small Business Administration for further information at http://www.sba.com.

Determining a Business Entity

Any occupational therapist functioning as an independent consultant, i.e., receives fee for services, is considered a business by the Internal Revenue Service (IRS). The OT must report any business incomes to the government. In doing this, a decision must be made about what business form the practice is to take and the steps initiated to establish it. There are three basic types of business organizations:

- Proprietorships
- Partnerships
- Corporations

Within these business forms, there are five versions to consider:

- Sole proprietorships
- Partnerships (general or limited)
- Corporations (C-Type)
- Corporations (S-Type)
- Limited liability corporations (LLC)

In determining an appropriate business entity, there are choices and repercussions and restrictions associated with each. There are guidelines and taxation differences to review. Because every practice is individual with varying needs, the reader is strongly recommended to seek advice from an accountant and lawyer prior to making this decision.

Local Licenses

One of the first steps after naming the business is to procure city and/or county business licenses and sales permits at city or county offices. There are usually fees for the initial applications, as well as for annual renewal of the licenses. Local licenses should be obtained before the business opens its doors to avoid fines. Depending upon the locale, businesses are taxed by the city or county, based on gross receipts or some other measure of productivity. City and state sales tax may be collected on products sold. Check with local government offices to determine the appropriate procedures for the area in question.

State Licenses

Some states have particular requirements for some professional businesses, such as education and experience requirements, examinations, detailed applications, or may require a fee to obtain a license to operate a business. The license is maintained by meeting that state's continuing education requirement (if any), and renewing the license periodically with an accompanying renewal fee. Consult an attorney and an accountant for this information.

This is not to be confused with the professional occupational therapy registration examination required by the National Board for Certification in Occupational Therapy, Inc. (NBCOT), www.nbcot.org/, or state licensure and certification. A majority of states require state licensing or certification of occupational therapists and occupational therapy assistants. If the state in which the practice is located has a license requirement, the steps for maintaining the license are the same as those described previously. It is important to get complete information on the specific requirements of the state in which the practice will be located.

State licensing and regulating agencies for individual states can be found in Appendix A-3.2.

Other resources to assist the entrepreneur are the Small Business Administration previously mentioned, and numerous books and web addresses. Hundreds of free resources and book profiles about operating a business can be located at www.smartbiz.com.

An overview of state and federal regulations, taxation, and business entities are described specific to each state in *Smart Starting Your Business In…* (available in titles for all states), by Jenkins (1996). More information can be obtained at www.smartbiz.com/sbs/books/book783.htm.

Tax Identification Numbers and IRS Requirements

Each person or corporation doing business in a state must submit a tax application form to the state's department of revenue, along with a registration fee. After registration, the state issues the business an identification number and sends out necessary tax forms (e.g., sales tax, state sales tax, payroll tax). As early as possible, the business should apply for a federal employer identification number (EIN). An EIN is used to identify the business for most federal tax purposes (e.g., payroll and income tax returns). An EIN is obtained by filing a completed *Form SS-4* entitled 0400 Application for Employer Identification Number. To request an EIN application by mail, dial 1-800-829-1040. To receive an EIN over the telephone or to mail an application, use the form number and address of the center for the state of interest in the appropriate Regional IRS Centers, by clicking on the appropriate state at www.irs.gov/where_file/

index.html. Allow four to five weeks if the application is done by mail. EINs can also be obtained over the phone, but there is a long distance charge for the call. Forms can be downloaded or received by fax. Visit the Internal Revenue Service at www.irs.gov/bus_info/library.html for the EIN application and many other IRS publications and forms. Among those of interest are *The IRS Tax Guide for Small Business*, 1999 publication 334, *Starting and Keeping Records*, Pub 583, and the Circular E *Employers Tax Guide* will also be of value to the private practitioner and will be found at this web address.

When hiring employees, the practice owner needs to provide the appropriate paperwork for new employees to complete, such as a W4 "Employees Withholding Certificate," an I9 "Employment Eligibility Verification," and a state income tax withholding form (the type of form varies depending on the state). Again, these forms can be obtained (with certain printing specifications) from the IRS website and the state department of revenue.

Monthly, quarterly, and or annual federal and state income tax withholding payments as well as FICA, Social Security and Medicare contributions for each employee must be made. The federal publication previously mentioned entitled Pub 15 Circular E *Employers Tax Guide*, and equivalent state publications will assist the employer in lawful business practices. It cannot be stressed strongly enough that an accountant should handle these complicated aspects of the business, unless the business owner has expertise in this area. The penalties are too high for mistakes in this area to take tax management lightly.

In addition, a state unemployment number must be received through the state's department of revenue and regular contributions made for each employee on a quarterly basis or as mandated by the state.

At the end of the calendar year, each employee must receive a W2 form by January 31, indicating the annual amount of income and withholding.

If hiring subcontractors, each individual must receive a 1099 at the end of the calendar year if they have been paid more than $500.00. Many accountants, however, recommend sending every subcontractor a 1099. Use of subcontractors requires some thought to assure that they would not be considered an employee by the state and federal government. In addition, as an independent practitioner or contractor, make sure to follow the same guidelines so that those you provide service to will have no question.

Stephen Fishman (2000) identifies the following "Ten Tips for Employers Who Hire Independent Contractors":

1. Use written agreements.
2. File all required 1099s.
3. Hire for specific tasks.
4. Obtain independent contractors' taxpayer ID numbers.
5. Don't supervise independent contractors.
6. Don't give free equipment and office space.
7. Require invoices.
8. Hire incorporated independent contractors.
9. Keep good records.
10. Understand copyright ownership rules.

Although these tips are not rules, there is often a gray area where subcontractors are concerned. It is better use a conservative approach in this regard because the fines imposed if a business is in violation are stiff. The IRS and the state departments of revenue view the use of subcontractors as a significant loss of tax dollars and would prefer that workers are hired as employees.

Space for Private Practice

There are three choices when considering space options for a private practice:

1. Free-standing office
2. In-home office
3. Other; mobile

Office Space—Free-Standing

Leased or purchased office space can be used for conducting an occupational therapy business. The location should be:

- Close to the medical community
- Conveniently located
- Served by adequate parking
- Accessible
- Noninclusive of similar businesses (no other OTs in the building)

A real estate agent can help to identify available space, properties, and trends for health care services in specific locations/geographical areas. Costs will vary, but other points when choosing appropriate office space are:

- Is there exposure to the community and general public?
- Does it comply with the ADA?
- Do zoning laws permit health care services there?
- Do the neighborhood businesses/practices enhance or detract from the OT services offered?
- Can a "right of first refusal" be negotiated in the lease? This will be important if planning for possible expansion someday. This allows the leasee to be the first to refuse neighboring space, should it become available.

It is important to seek professional advice when making decisions about leasing or buying, to determine its effect on the tax situation of a new practice. For more information about planning and space requirements, see Chapter 1.

In-home Office

For tax purposes, the IRS has regulated what is actually considered a home office. To receive a deduction for home office when filing income tax returns, there are a number of considerations, as mentioned in IRS Publication 587, *Business Use of Your Home*, www.irs.gov/bus_info/library.html.

The IRS Publication states that the area used for business must be used "regularly" and "exclusively": 1) as the principal place of business (including administrative use), 2) as a place to meet or deal with clients in the normal course of the business, or 3) in connection with the business if it is a separate structure not attached to the taxpayer's personal residence. If servicing consumers from a home office, there are considerations related to zoning, parking, public restrooms, signage, and accessibility compliance issues to be aware of. Medicare and other reimbursement sources may not acknowledge a home office setting. Restrictions also may exist in the individual home title. Checking Americans with Disabilities Act (ADA) regulations, city and county ordinances, title companies, and reimbursement sources prior to establishing a home office is recommended.

If one does qualify for a home office, the business expenses below are generally deductible on IRS Form 8829 as reported by in the IRS Pub 587 as a percentage of:

- Real estate tax
- Homeowner's insurance
- Utilities
- Mortgage interest
- Home repairs/maintenance
- Security system
- Rent
- Depreciation
- Casualty losses
- Other: water, sewer, garbage removal, snow plowing, etc.

The business percentage of the home is determined by dividing the area exclusively used for business by the total area of the house, with some exclusions.

Direct expenses are generally 100 percent deductible against business income. This includes repairs and painting/remodeling made to the specific area or room used specifically for business.

Indirect expenses are the upkeep and running of the entire home. The business percent of indirect expenses is generally deductible against business income. This percentage may differ from the percentage calculated in Part 1 of Form 8829. Always check the IRS publication 587 and/or consult with an accountant prior to filing a deduction for home office use.

Other

Some types of occupational therapy practice do not require space, therefore, significantly reduce the amount of overhead expense required to operate the practice. Providing services in sheltered workshops, consumer's home, school settings, businesses and industry, medical facilities, wellness centers, etc. may eliminate the need for actual clinic space. In this case, the therapist must learn to organize equipment, supplies, paperwork, and schedule in a method that is portable and transitional.

Naming the Practice

Selecting an appropriate name for any occupational therapy practice can be a marketing tool in itself. The name of the practice can communicate the types of services offered, the location of the business, how services are provided, and to whom they are provided. It can also create a desired image, or reflect negatively if chosen poorly.

A professional practice should avoid confusing or whimsical names that may "turn off" the market. "Get a Grip Hand Therapy" is original and humorous but may be perceived as unprofessional by some. "Functional Improvement Center" is clear to rehabilitation professionals, but could be confusing to the general public.

The alphabetical listing of a name is also a consideration, according to some small business consultants, as the consumer may choose it more frequently if it is presented first in the yellow pages. Avoid use of common or generic wording in the business name, to protect a company name from legal use by others.

Research is important to assure the chosen practice name is not protected by a trademark under state or federal law. Check the annual publication *The Trademark Register* at the library or on the Internet to confirm absence of conflict with a registered trade name. An initial error in this area can be costly and devastating to a new business due to trademark infringement. Trademark Scan is an on-line search updated weekly or bi-weekly, containing comprehensive information on the names of trademarks registered federally in all fifty states and in Puerto Rico (www.pmal.fplc.edu/ipcorner/bp99/paper2.htm). "So You Wanna Register a Trademark?" website provides good information on the process of trademark registration and search, while giving the viewer link options to other sites, and can be found at www.soyouwanna.com/site/syws/trademark/trademarkFULL.html. Other scanning services are available to the future business owner, which include but are not limited to: www.nameprotect.com/freemon.html offering free scanning and name registration, and www.register.com/, which is used to search for duplicate website names.

A good name is simple, spellable, memorable, and has dignity (McCollom & Mynders, 1984). A practice may benefit from being named after the owner, but it may pose difficulty when selling a practice to a new owner with a different name. Difficult personal names are not recommended. Incorporating a street or geographical name into the practice name clarifies location, however, it may cause confusion should the business choose to move in the future.

Business Office Management

An efficient and profitable business can only be achieved with competent business management staff. Billing, transcription, and reception services are critical for the life of a therapy practice. Contracting with businesses specializing in billing and transcription services may be an alternative to in-house employees. This option can be beneficial in many ways:

- Saves space (work is performed at contractor's office)
- Less overhead expense (no tax burden associated with employees, no start-up costs related to equipment)
- Efficiency and competency in work; paid on revenues received or pages typed
- No initial financial investment

Negatives to hiring subcontractors to perform office work include:

- More costly at times over extended period
- Receptionist may still be required and computer at the office may still be necessary
- Lack of control over work performed

If the business owner chooses to have these duties performed "in-house," the following considerations exist:

- Billing software. A wide variety of choices with a range in expense from ($1,000 to $5,000) and function (scheduling, voicing, and billing) are available.
- Space and equipment expense. See Chapter 1 for choosing space and equipment for the office needs.
- Competence in OT billing using Current Procedural Terminology (CPT) coding, invoicing, and cash collections. For profits to be realized, correct coding and billing procedures must be followed. It is incumbent on the provider to follow ethical billing procedures, and keep informed about

changes in reimbursement policies and legislation. Ignorance is not an acceptable excuse for billing mistakes if legal issues arise. For more detailed information regarding reimbursement issues, see Chapter 6.

- A receptionist in the office is a luxury many cannot initially afford. Voice mail systems have become more acceptable and thorough, and therefore, can suffice temporarily. A receptionist is invaluable, however, in a busy office to organize the schedule, phone calls, and paperwork for therapists. Hiring a person for this position may become a priority as the business grows.

In organizing the management of the office systems, it is recommended that an accountant be consulted and in many cases used regularly to set up and maintain the books. Good advice and guidance by an accountant can save time, money, and problems in the long run.

Summary

If starting a private practice is correctly implemented, the risks can be outweighed by the benefits of being self-employed. For a successful private practice to exist, the owner/manager must be willing to invest a significant amount of time, and possibly money in the venture, initially. Persevering through the ups and downs will ensure longevity, if positive decisions are made.

With careful and meticulous planning, a vision for the future, and a proactive marketing approach, the private practitioner can build a secure foundation for the services OTs can deliver, now and into the future.

Case Study 1

An OT entrepreneur is interested in opening a pediatric clinic in the state of North Carolina with the name Child Development Center of Ashville.

Discussion Questions

1. Is the name of the practice available?
2. What regional IRS center needs to be contacted to obtain an EIN number?

Group Project

Develop a practice model for a private therapy business. Include the following information and present the model to an audience:

1. Projected budget
2. One and three year projections for revenue and expenses
3. List of start-up items including expenses
4. Sample business plan
5. Application for EIN number
6. Determination of business entity

CHAPTER 4

Leadership and Staff Management

By Barbara Broadbridge

Good leadership skills are essential to maintain a high level of staff satisfaction, productivity, and cohesiveness. When the strengths of employees are promoted, job satisfaction, as well as therapy services, will grow. The opposite effect can be seen, however, when a therapist is stifled by lack of empowerment. Frustration and stagnation should not be allowed to suffocate enthusiasm and team contribution.

The employee should be considered an internal customer to the manager. The internal customer must be treated with respect and dignity. By helping to engage staff in reaching their full potential, the manager successfully fills his or her role as a supervisor. (For purposes of this chapter the terms manager, leader, and supervisor will be used interchangeably.)

Offering feedback about employee performance is part of the manager's role. Methods of completing this include, but are not limited to, performance reviews and face to face contact. Sometimes this requires disciplinary plans and actions, and at times may result in termination. Good leadership skills are essential for positive results to occur from any of these and other supervisory duties.

At the conclusion of this chapter, the reader will be able to:

1. Understand the role of a supervisor.

2. Establish a frame of reference for the core values of a good leader.

3. Deal with employee morale and conflict resolution issues.

4. Perform a performance review and guide the employee in goal setting.

5. Determine guidelines for disciplinary action and termination of employees.

6. List methods of providing feedback about performance and reinforcement for positive results.

Leadership Techniques

Therapy programs and practices, like all businesses, succeed or fail because of the people involved. A successful leader retains and motivates people, the company's most valuable asset.

One of the key success factors for a health care business is the ability to retain employees, and one of the most important factors in employee job satisfaction is their supervisor's style of management. Countless surveys have been conducted regarding job satisfaction. While most people assume that "salary" would rank high, it does not. Money can attract people to a job but it typically does not keep them there.

Core Values

Establishing the "core values" of respect, dignity, confidentiality, support, and honesty will retain employees. They are essential characteristics in an effective leader. Good leaders handle their internal customers (employees) as carefully as they handle their external customers (consumers).

In addition to core values, effective leaders must develop a wide variety of management skills. Clinical practice leaders must be detail oriented while seeing the whole picture. In addition, clinical practice leaders should remember the following:

- They must coach and remove barriers for clinicians while serving as clinical mentors in their areas of expertise.
- They must know how to delegate and more importantly follow up on assignments.
- They must be able to motivate a team to pursue and exceed the organization's goals.
- They are patient advocates, committed to improving quality and providing exceptional customer service.
- Exceptional leaders will embrace change while providing stability for their team.
- They will get results by leading and motivating their team.
- Most importantly, effective leaders are ethical leaders.

Successful leaders have a deep seated belief that all employees deserve their respect. A leader does not always have to agree or understand an employee to treat them respectfully. Employees want to rely on the integrity of their supervisor. Trust must be earned from every employee; it is a slow process and trust is almost impossible to earn back a second time.

Managers must be consistently honest and up-front with their employees. There are frequently times in a manager's duties when it is inappropriate to share information with employees for corporate or legal reasons. It is at these times that a manager must choose his or her words wisely, seeking advice from superiors or mentors, or other individuals who offer professional support, guidance, instruction, and role modeling to bring an employee to their maximum potential. While confidentiality is an assumed "common sense" skill for a clinician, it can be challenging as a supervisor. It is lonely at the top and there is a natural need to express issues to someone else (otherwise known as venting) as they arise.

Employees will trust a manager who is predictable, consistent, and admits mistakes. Being able to listen and truly hear opinions that are different from one's own is an important managerial skill when supervising a diverse work group. Although it can be tough to work closely with individuals who have opposite viewpoints or working styles, the rewards can be many for consumers.

Just as consumers are different, so are employees, and their preferred styles vary. Strive to value diversity. Respect the differences of others through actions and words, and the program or practice will be respected.

Morale

Employees do not come to work to make mistakes. They are generally full of hope and excitement when they accept a job. It is the job of a supervisor to keep that fire alive in an employee. Do this by finding out what gets them enthusiastic and help them avoid burnout. This can be done through feedback and reinforcement.

Feedback and Reinforcement

No one minds a pat on the back for a job well done, or words of appreciation for their dedication. Ask ten people if they would like receiving more positive feedback at work and the vast majority will say yes. This employee benefit will not cost a company a dime and the rewards in employee retention are well documented.

There is little risk in giving too much feedback. On the reverse side, no one wants to be the last to know they are making errors. Telling an employee up front and in a timely manner what they are doing well and, constructively, what should be changed about their performance will result in more of the desired behavior and less of the undesired behavior. Be specific and sincere. Use examples and propose solutions. Do not wait for a gold medal performance to recognize your internal customers. Commit to making constructive feedback a daily habit.

Frequently managers get pulled away from their responsibilities to employees by other crises, deadlines, or a single problem employee. Managers find themselves giving all their time to problems, while unintentionally ignoring the great clinicians that are working for them. Schedule time in your calendar to have one-on-one meetings with employees and be sure to reschedule those that are missed. Make these contacts with the internal customer a priority. Send weekly thank you notes or leave "you're appreciated" voice mails for staff. Other small gestures may include but are not limited to the occasional card, phone call, award recognition, coffee, lunch, dessert, pizza party, gift certificate, or even a financial bonus, if feasible. Although these efforts can be quickly overlooked when swamped with work or under stress, chances are many of the same problems bothering the manager may be affecting the employee. The quick note or gesture given can make a real difference in employee morale.

Communication

Another critical skill for successful leaders is the ability to communicate effectively. Let employees know what is going on. They want to feel included. Make them feel important through communicating with them regularly and soliciting their feedback.

Communicate regularly and consistently, not just when big issues arise. Practice this skill at the beginning of the employee/employer relationship. If employees have only seen their manager when problems arise, their presence will be dreaded and feared. A manager's nightmare is to be associated only with bad news, which can put the manager at a large disadvantage when trying to deliver a message in the most positive light.

Even if there is no agenda and nothing to share, "manage by walking around" and see what employees have to say. Get to know the staff and its dynamics. The better the employees and their need, are understood, the better they can be served.

Let them know the door is always open to them. This does not mean they can walk in at any time. It means that there is always time in the schedule for them, because they are valued. An employee who feels respected and taken care of at work does a much better job with the consumers than a disgruntled employee.

Growth Through Staff Ownership and Satisfaction

Although job satisfaction among staff is necessary to add new services, it may also be encouraged by giving employee(s) ownership for programs, promoting new educational opportunities, or by tapping into individual resources. A manager who overlooks an employee's enthusiasm and interest in learning, or who channels staff indefinitely into areas of non-interest, may find poor employee morale, lack of loyalty, or apathetic work behaviors. Job satisfaction is the catalyst to staff stability and forward progress in the department. If input is consistently requested from staff about program changes and additions, the employees' feeling of ownership for their work is promoted while strengthening the growth potential of the department.

Often, therapists' interest and experience guide the OT manager in appropriate paths of program development. Other times, community need dictates services to be offered. In either case, a visionary leader/manager will capitalize on opportunities to establish new programs and create a climate of employee empowerment.

Employee Retention

Motivating staff, preventing burnout, and stopping employee turnover must be a priority at *all* times, not just when problems arise. Proactively ask individual employees what they like and dislike about their job. Sometimes employees will open up more in a group setting, but give them the opportunity for one-on-one time as well, to really get to know them. Insist that they provide potential solutions with all issues, but be there to give advice when they cannot see past the problem.

Remember to celebrate small successes and have some fun at work. Start traditions that employees look forward to in the future. Plan ahead to celebrate significant consumer progress with consumers and their families. When successful surveys are completed (e.g., Joint Commission on Accreditation of Healthcare Organizations or Medicare), host an employee luncheon for their efforts. Get employees excited when patient satisfaction surveys or outcomes improve, or when the practice obtains a new contract or referral source. Again, do not wait for the "100th" anniversary of the practice to celebrate with the program.

Flexiblity and Creativity

Creative thinking is needed to retain employees when clinical jobs are plentiful. As stated earlier in this chapter, money is not going to retain employees. Things like flexibility can be far more valuable to working parents or clinicians. Long-term commitments are frequently gained from current staff by asking them to propose a better schedule for themselves. It may take some work to accommodate the schedule, but the payoff is high.

Managing Proactively

Be committed to providing the team a consistent foundation regarding the philosophy, policies and procedures, and goals of the organization. Foster success and accountability in every employee through orientation. Timely and effective orientation is important in the retention of new employees. Make sure the "new hire" completely understands the expectations of the job, their job description, and performance indicators. Very importantly, make it clear what violations prompt immediate dismissal. Document and have all parties sign evidence of this information being provided.

After the probationary period (usually three to six months), supervisors should support an ongoing professional development plan for each employee. The plans can include clinical mentoring, formal or informal continuing education, and opportunities to work with new diagnoses. Time spent early in the relationship on formal coaching to improve knowledge, skills, or behavior is well invested. Informal coaching through spontaneous praise or recognition will also build confidence in employees.

Job Satisfaction

Retention and employee satisfaction do not necessarily go hand-in-hand, and job satisfaction is not the opposite of job dissatisfaction. As an example, supervisor dishonesty can make an employee leave; but supervisor honesty is expected, and will not make them stay. Motivating, offering challenging work, and fostering a feeling of worth combined with placing the employee in a position that is compatible with his or her personal life is a good start. If asked often enough, employees will discuss what job factors will retain them. The only thing worse than having a good employee leave a department is having an unhappy employee stay. They drag down other employees and do not represent the service well to customers. Let employees know that mediocre performance is not acceptable. Negative attitudes can be very contagious and affect morale of other staff.

Money can attract a clinician to a job but it will not keep them there. Sometimes employees take a job with the primary reason of getting out of their current job. They must feel valued, challenged, and supported if they are going to remain at a job.

Just as the employee's goals and objectives are regularly addressed, so should their job satisfaction. Ask them exactly what will make them stay with the organization and what issues have ever caused them to consider leaving. Retention and employee satisfaction cannot truly be addressed until these answers have been obtained from every employee. Only then will managers and supervisors know where to focus their attention.

The following key concepts should be reviewed when assessing job satisfaction.

1. Staff reinforcement—Verbal recognition for work performed should include supervisor feedback, as well as goal setting for consistent, positive feedback. Small gestures of appreciation, may include but are not limited to the occasional card, phone call, note, award, coffee, lunch, dessert, pizza party, gift certificate, or financial bonus.

2. Employee appraisals—A written measurement of work performed should be completed annually. Specific tasks of the job need to be identified and objective feedback given as related to work completed. Allow employee to appraise self, as well as the manager's supervisory skills.

3. Salary, pay increases—Annual reviews and raises are more effective as a reinforcement if there is a correlation between them. In other words, they are offered in recognition of good work performed. Automatic annual pay increases become expected and decrease worker motivation to improve performance. Financial rewards that are competitive to the employment market are most useful.

4. Benefits—Many types of fringe benefit programs are possible. A paid time off system offering vacation, sick leave, holidays, funeral leave, and/or personal leave is a plus. Dues for association memberships and certification fees are optional. When offered, professional membership benefits add professionalism to the entire program through publications received and continuing education opportunities and discounts. Political action is indirectly supported by requiring staff to be members of state and national associations. A liberal continuing education program is recommended to promote learning and program growth. Retirement plans, 401-K, and tax sheltered annuities are common inclusions.

5. Flexible hours—Use of variable scheduling, 10 hour days, split shifts, early or late hours is helpful for the consumer, as well as the employee at times. Finding a compatible time table for employees can increase quality and productivity by utilizing the employee's hours of maximum effectiveness.

6. Part-time options—Job sharing and part-time positions provide opportunities to balance home life with career ambitions. Some employers reduce or eliminate benefits for part-time workers, which reduces the overhead burden for the company.

7. Opportunity for advancement—Some employees aspire to hold leadership positions or contribute at greater levels within the department. Reinforcing these efforts through additional responsibility can create empowerment and program ownership.

8. Cohesive work environment—Encourage positive inter/intradepartmental relationships through modeling, communication, and team building. Using a no tolerance approach to nonproductive and destructive interactions among staff is an important precedent. Dealing with issues openly as they arise may curtail unresolved issues.

9. Professionally challenging position—Apathy and complacency can destroy a good employee. Be aware of this possibility and challenge employees to strive for excellence and professional growth. Allow staff to develop programs, take courses, and attend continuing education seminars regularly.

10. Job security—Feeling unsure about the stability of one's position creates anxiety and undue stress, often interfering in contentment. If job instability exists, be emotionally supportive and honest about the situation. The staff member who feels part of the mission of the department will respond as if it were "their" program and not merely the owner's/manager's.

11. Ability to be involved in political issues regarding OT—Allow and even encourage staff to hold committee, board, or active membership positions in the profession. This may require use of some of the department's resources such as paper, copies, postage, and staff time (if approved). However, the benefits to OT and visibility among colleagues is a great asset.

12. Membership in community service organizations—Offering time off for attendance at community service group meetings, (e.g., Kiwanis, Rotary, Lions, Optimists Clubs) as well as paying for membership dues can be a positive optional benefit for an employee as well as the community. This can also prove to be an effective marketing tool for community and business awareness of occupational therapy.

Affects of Attrition and Worker Overload on Morale and Department Expansion

Employee attrition is a natural part of personnel management, although attempting to keep attrition at a minimum is encouraged. Replacing staff can be costly, as well as disruptive to the cohesion and progress of the occupational therapy department. The dynamics of a group change when an employee leaves. There is an adjustment to new personalities when an open position is filled. Any momentum previously experienced may be delayed. If the position is not filled immediately, the level of stress may increase within the department due to added workloads. Filling the gap may be difficult but it is important to continue high quality consumer services, even if a waiting list or overtime is necessary.

It may take a period of several months to experience a boost in momentum and morale following a change in staff, even when a change means adding a new position. A new personality in the crowd can spark a "honeymoon effect": the first several months are a dynamic high, with energies plummeting sometime in the near future. Open staff communication regarding roles, restructuring, and responsibilities will direct changes with the least resistance.

Participatory planning sparks ownership and self-motivation while creating group cohesion. When long-term work overload exists, the possibility of staff burnout increases. This factor has the potential to multiply problems and may lead to further attrition. Reinforcements at this level are critical, as mentioned previously in this chapter. Acknowledgement of the situation and participatory leadership (e.g., manager engaging in hands-on assistance with caseload) will demonstrate understanding while fostering respect.

Maintaining balance among co-workers reduces burnout, conflict, and work related stressors. When the caseload is high, this is not always possible. Therefore, efforts should be made whenever possible to:

- Equalize workload ratios to hours worked. For example, if Sue works 40 hours/week and Bill works 20 hours/week and they are both 60 percent productive, then Sue will treat consumers 24 hours/week and Bill 12.
- Implement fair and liberal time off policies for personal/family matters, within the limits of meeting caseload needs.
- Reinforce open and positive communication among workers/co-workers.
- Reward efforts to collaborate with team members for the benefit of the consumer.
- Model respectful attitudes/behaviors toward others.
- Schedule paperwork time into daily schedule to eliminate the need to take work home.
- If caseload warrants a need to cut employees' hours, do so as equitably as possible. Offer voluntary "low census" (non-paid time off based on reduced consumer load).

Conflict Resolution

A smart leader lets his or her teams know it is acceptable to disagree. As long as individuals disagree in an appropriate manner, at the right place, and to the right person, it can be very beneficial to the practice.

Complaining and moaning behind the scenes accomplishes nothing. Managers should instill a "fix it or move on" attitude. Conflict resolution can be healthy when the focus is finding the best solution. It can be destructive, however, when the focus is on winning at all costs.

Conflicts arise when employees have different interpretations or priorities. These differences can sometimes be resolved through better communication. Start by listening to uncover the real problems. Leaders strive for win/win solutions. Keep the conflict about *ideas* not individuals. Start the bridge-building process by restating areas of agreement before dealing with the disagreement.

Managers who surround themselves with "yes" people are ineffective leaders. Terminating a "trouble maker" is not always better for the harmony of a group; there will always be challenging personalities in a group. The stronger an employee is, the more likely it is that they will criticize decisions and possibly cause turmoil. It is natural for independent, creative thinkers to question authority and as long as it is constructive and appropriate, the manager should welcome the challenge.

Difficult circumstances, tough choices, and hard decisions build character. A manager's positive response to criticism can improve relationships and enhance his or her image as a leader. A good leader will respond to criticism with interest rather than fear or resentment. If feedback is not presented constructively, it can still be an opportunity for growth. The best way to learn how one is perceived is by listening to criticism, constructive or not. A manager can be *receptive* to negative feedback without necessarily *agreeing* with it.

Do not define team players as employees that do not "rock the boat," question, or step out of line. Create a culture where it is acceptable to disagree and question, and employees will feel able to vent and channel their grievances through managers and supervisors. This reduces the amount of negative and destructive comments and venting done among the team.

Listen, but be careful not to step in when differences should be worked out among employees. Conflicts do not always need a referee. Good leaders uncover the real reasons for grievances and ask disruptive people for their help. Consider putting together a problem solving team. The team must first achieve mutual understanding of the problem, which is half the battle. They then outline and examine all options as a group, before coming to a decision. Only when disruptions outweigh employee contributions and become destructive should disciplinary action steps be taken.

Managers need to take steps to keep their own motivation and job satisfaction high during conflicts. Take time to get focused when the job gets tough. Articulate the big picture to employees during times of stress. Communicate your expectations that all employees establish and maintain healthy interpersonal relationships with each other. Relationships should be equally respectful, regardless of job title or educational degree. Remind employees that human errors are opportunities for forgiveness and growth, not for shame and guilt. Adopt a no tolerance approach to destructive worker behaviors amongst the team. Be consistent and address problems before they get out of proportion. Employees need to be expected to treat each other, including the manager, with the same core values discussed earlier.

A person in authority should assume the attitude of a servant to the internal customer; remembering that helping others resolve conflicts and achieve success is a great occupation with many rewards.

Performance Reviews

Be candid about performance expectations with every new clinician. Establishing performance guidelines at the beginning of employment helps lay the foundation for a long-term, mutually beneficial relationship. A proper, respectful performance review is not only conducted at the employee's one-year anniversary or on an annual basis, but feedback should be offered frequently and consistently.

Goals

Performance reviews should be *ongoing* and based on goals set up front. Objective performance indicators measure achievement of agreed upon goals. Managers should collect external benchmarking information, factoring in variations like facility size or marketplace differences. There should be standard measures for all employees. For an example of a employee goal sheet/action plan, which can also be used for a disciplinary action plan, see Figure 4.1. Statistics and data should be shared openly and frequently to give employees ongoing opportunities to make adjustments or seek assistance if necessary. Address issues proactively and while they are still minor.

Early careerists may require weekly or biweekly meetings regarding their work, where monthly meetings may be appropriate for middle managers or senior clinicians. These meetings should give both parties the opportunity to address needs. The meetings can be in person or by phone but should be private and scheduled in advance. Documented regular discussions about workload, goals, and recommended adjustments should then be compiled for quarterly reviews. All of this information can be rolled into an annual review at potential raise time, but there should be no surprises in the annual review. Waiting one year to tell an internal customer that you are not satisfied with an aspect of their work is not only an outdated practice, it is disrespectful. Open, honest, up-front communication is what will make relationships strong and the practice succeed.

Employees will only change their behavior if they know they need to. Employees who are headed in the right direction will second guess themselves only when given inadequate guidance and support. Tell them and tell them frequently what you expect and when they are delivering.

Performance Indicators

Clinicians need to understand that clinical competencies are not the only factors being judged by the employer. All performance criteria should be written out and should be consistent with the job description.

Typical areas for reviewing clinicians include:

- Written and oral communication skills
- Teaching skills
- Teamwork
- Customer service
- Patient advocacy
- Flexibility
- Time management and productivity
- Organizational skills

PAGE ____ of ____

PROFESSIONAL GOAL SHEET AND ACTION PLAN

Employee _____

Department _____

PERFORMANCE OBJECTIVE	RESPONSIBLE PARTIES	TARGET DATE	EXPECTED OUTCOME	ACTUAL OUTCOME	INITIALS

Figure 4.1. Professional Goal Sheet and Action Plan

- Clinical problem solving skills
- Ability to optimize the functional abilities of patients
- Clinical competencies specific to the job

Let clinicians know that ownership for showing accomplishments and progress throughout the entire year rests with them. Just like performance reviews, tracking progress towards goals should be ongoing and not an annual event. A good employee will answer the question "How well did you perform your job this year?" for the employer. A great employee will answer the question "How did you improve your job?" for the employer. Performance reviews should be objective. The employee should have documentation of progress towards their professional goals. A formal peer review system is strongly encouraged to give employees continuous feedback on the content quality, clarity, and completeness of their documentation. Patient satisfaction surveys can be utilized to review customer service skills.

Conducting the Performance Review

Most managers dread the actual face-to-face performance review because they do all the talking and they fear potential employee reactions. During a proper performance review, the employee should do the majority of the talking. Since strengths and weaknesses have been discussed throughout the year, they are not the focus of the meeting. They are reviewed, but the bulk of the meeting is focused on adjusting goals for the future and having the clinician take ownership of the action plan.

In addition, the supervisor should commit to resolving any company roadblocks prohibiting the clinician's success. A partnership should be developed. There should be no big reactions because there will be no big surprises. If conducted properly, the meeting should not be dreaded. It should be uplifting and encouraging.

Supervisors should never "wing" or rush a performance review. Both the formal review and an agenda should be written out ahead of time with space left open to add the action plan developed during the meeting. Employees should be given proper notice in order to prepare for the meeting.

First, recognize accomplishments and discuss the employee's potential. Ask the employee about obstacles and solutions, reiterating that responsibility for improvement remains with the employee. Continue asking open-ended questions until the clinician addresses all issues and proposes appropriate solutions for each one. Mutually agree upon solutions to each problem and put them in writing. Then encourage and support the employee's plan, always ending the review on a positive note. Proper performance reviews will help build trust, instill confidence, and inspire higher performance.

See Figure 4.2 for a sample performance review form.

Disciplinary Action

When considering the termination of an employee, a manager must make sure all avenues for improvement have been exhausted. Disciplinary action is designed to communicate clearly in a progressive manner and give every employee a fair chance to improve his or her performance.

Frequent display of poor performance is a result of poor communication and usually can be fixed. When this is the case, and the employee makes the

Performance Review Form

Employee:
Date of Review:
Date of Hire:

RATING SCALE:

Always	5
Almost always (75%)	4
Usually (50%)	3
Needs improvement (25%)	2
Continues to need improvement	1*
Unacceptable (never)	0*

*will be addressed in attached goal sheet with action plan

Performance areas	Ability to perform duties of the job	Rating
Takes initiative and responsibility for duties		
Is timely in attendance to work and for appointments		
Completes paperwork requirements thoroughly and on a timely basis		
Stays on schedule, acknowledges patients if delayed		
Notifies supervisor in timely manner if unable to attend work		
Handles workload with confidence and ease		
Accepts supervision		
Follows policies and procedures		
Handles feedback positively		
Provides direction and supervision to others as needed		

Figure 4.2. Sample Performance Review form *(continues)*

Performance areas	Ability to perform duties of the job	Rating
Supervises co-workers and students appropriately		
Clearly communicates instructions and intentions to patients		
Implements accurate, thorough, and skilled OT		
Takes initiative to study unfamiliar treatment techniques and procedures		
Communicates effectively with patients, supervisor, and co-workers		
Resolves conflict issues appropriately		
Presents self professionally to others in dress, body language, and overt expression		
Treats patients with compassion, helps patients to feel confidence in therapy		
Accepts other duties as assigned with a positive attitude		
Additional Comments: (attach copy of goal sheet)		

_____
Employee Signature

_____
Manager Signature

Figure 4.2. Sample Performance Review form *(continued)*

requested changes, be careful not to slip back into the old communication style once the issues are resolved. This creates a situation where time is spent with an employee fluctuating between disciplinary action and average performance throughout the year.

When disciplinary action is considered, decide if the employee cannot do the job, or *will not* do the job. Always examine the *problem* not the *person*. Unfortunately, some jobs do not fit for some people and no amount of coaching can rectify the situation. Although the employee may be a good person, the job may not be a match for their skills or style.

Documentation is the key to fair disciplinary action. This enables both parties to see clear expectations and consequences with little room for misinterpretation. Figure 4.1 shows how an employee goal sheet can be used for a disciplinary action plan.

When disciplinary action becomes necessary, consider the rules of thumb listed below:

- Disciplinary action plans should contain an outline of each performance issue separately.

- Each issue should have examples and recommendations to correct each problem, as well as target dates to achieve each recommendation.

- Give *specific* past examples.

- Focus on future expectations.

- Focus on *behaviors*, not attitudes.

- Be sure the performance areas addressed are compatible to the information on previous performance reviews.

- If an employee cries or "blows up" during the meeting, wait quietly for them to compose themselves before continuing.

- If a union contract requires that a union representative be present during performance discussions, comply; but always direct any communication to the employee.

- Have employee set an action plan for expected improvements (Figure 4.1).

- Both parties must sign and retain copies of the established plan.

- Always document the meeting and commitments made by both parties and attach a copy of the disciplinary action plan.

It is important to note that employees must perceive that the disciplinary action is in their best interest. They must accept that the changes are necessary, or the disciplinary plan is likely to fail. A higher success rate will be achieved if the employee comes up with the solutions and assists in setting the deadlines. Use open-ended questions to draw solutions out of a clinician, especially if it is apparent that they are waiting to receive direction from the manager. Ask them what obstacles exist that might not be overtly apparent.

Follow up again at a preestablished time to ensure that proper progress is being made in the employee's performance. Make certain to acknowledge any improved behavior as it occurs, as well as during follow up meetings. Timely follow up is essential to the long-term success of the relationship. Often, due to other managerial priorities, follow up is only completed on a timely basis when things are *not* going well. This trap should be avoided because it portrays the wrong message to a key contributor in the success of the practice—the employee.

Employee Terminations

Termination of an employee should not be considered unless the employee knows they are not meeting the expectations of the position, and all possible remedies have been tried and documented. Once it has been determined that an employee must be terminated due to poor performance, a quick resolution is advised. Having a disgruntled employee around the customers and other employees, even briefly, can cause great set backs in a program.

Schedule a termination meeting in a private setting, mid-afternoon, when no customers are nearby. This allows the terminated employee time to clear out their things while minimizing distractions to other workers. If there are any reasons to believe the employee may become threatening, plan ahead to have other managers or security close at hand. Position yourself close to the exit. Typically a sense of how the employee will react can be gathered from the disciplinary action sessions, unless there has been a severe violation requiring immediate termination.

Out of respect for the employee, terminations are typically done behind closed doors, one-on-one. If an employee has given a manager any reason to be concerned about their safety, leave the door cracked open, have an intercom system on, or have another manager in the room. While some employees get extremely angry when faced with termination, others will break down or try to negotiate their position back. The manager should anticipate their reaction but also be prepared to be surprised. We all react differently under severe stress and it is critical for the manager to anticipate and control their reactions as well. Being the terminator is just as stressful as being terminated.

Because it should have been made clear to employees upon hire what violations will result in immediate termination this documentation will support the case for termination if necessary. Do not assume the obvious is obvious to everyone. If this information was made available as part of the new employee orientation, then legal problems at time of termination will have been avoided. Make sure everything is properly documented, and obtain any needed approvals before terminating an employee. If there is any question, legal counsel should be consulted to eliminate legal risks associated with unlawful termination.

Termination for poor performance should never be a surprise. While documenting the failure to attain agreed upon goals or perform assigned tasks is challenging, documenting how subtle factors like "attitude" affect this person's ability to perform his or her job is extremely difficult. Be very careful to document valid reasons and hard facts for terminations. Laws protect employees, and ethical managers should not jeopardize the livelihood of employees based on emotions.

Conducting the Termination Meeting

It is a good idea to have a script to follow and role play the event in advance. Having remarks penciled out ahead of time will prevent the leader from getting drawn into a debate. The time for clarifications and negotiations was during the disciplinary action phase, not during the termination meeting.

In the meeting:

- Invite the employee to sit down. Then get right to the point.
- Simply state the fact that they are being terminated due to specific cause or causes, effective starting on specific date or time.
- Do not be apologetic or engage in small talk.

- Do not defend or justify the termination and do not let the meeting drag on.

- Give them a written list of company property that needs to be returned, e.g., keys, phone card, computer, patient files, equipment, reference books, cell phone, and pager.

- Let them know when to expect their final paycheck and if they are eligible for vacation payout or COBRA. COBRA allows them to be covered under the employer's health insurance policy, at their own expense, for a period of time based on a number of variables. They may be eligible to purchase disability, health, life, and dental insurance at the ex-employer's group rate from six to eighteen months, minimum. If they are, let them know when to expect mailings and give them a number to call if they have questions. If they are not eligible for insurance continuation, let them know their last date of coverage.

A common reason for clinicians being fired is because they are behind in their documentation. It is strongly advised that unless the clinician is a risk to patients, arrangements are made during the disciplinary action phase for the clinician to catch up and turn in all their patient documentation. You may even consider pulling them from consumer contact until they are caught up. Missing documentation from a terminated employee can turn into a serious problem.

Terminating an Employee Due to a Lay-off

The type of brief, factual meeting described above is not appropriate if an employee is being laid off due to reasons beyond their control. If someone's position has been eliminated, they should be allowed some time to absorb and process the news. They will typically go through all the emotions associated with any kind of loss. Supervisors feel worse knowing the employee did nothing to deserve this termination. Be careful to not make promises that cannot be kept and do not try to minimize the situation or offer false hopes. If an Employee Assistance Program or outplacement services are available, remind the employee of their purpose and potential benefit.

When someone is laid off, managers may want to consider not having them work during the paid notice period and let them leave early with pay. Give them a few days to say their goodbyes. However, for the remaining employee's sakes, do not let the transition drag on for long. They typically feel guilty that they still have a job, and the focus is definitely not on the consumers during this transition.

Communicating Terminations to Staff and Consumers

It is important for a supervisor to preplan how the termination will be communicated, after the fact, to internal and external customers. This step is one of the most critical and particularly hard in a practice that typically has open, honest communication. The manager is obligated to maintain confidentiality, out of respect for the terminated employee, and to avoid legal ramifications. However, loyalties should exist to the team that is staying. Morale can be significantly affected if the ex-employee was close to his or her co-workers.

Terminated employees do not usually tell both sides of the story on their way out the door. Be prepared to do damage control. Make it clear to other clinicians that the details of the employee's termination are confidential and that employees in the organization will never be surprised if their performance is not meeting expectations. Remind them of the progressive disciplinary action policy and the reasons for immediate termination.

If the termination was a lay-off there is a need to spend considerably more time with the remaining team members, both in a group setting and individually. Be honest with them about the stability of their jobs and the company. Point out all the positive steps they can take to secure their future, whether that is with this company or another. The bottom line, whether you have to terminate someone for poor performance or eliminate one position to salvage the rest, is to stick to your core values. Be fair, open, honest, and consistent, and have the documentation to prove it.

Summary

Although the challenges of being a department or team leader may not appeal to everyone, these positions can offer diverse opportunities in the area of administration. There are additional skills required of the supervisor that are not expected of the staff occupational therapist. The essence of leadership, however, is the same as that of dealing directly with the consumer. Guiding individuals to reach their maximum functional potential and achieve their goals in established performance areas are among the tasks that both the staff OT and the department leader(s) have in common.

Case Study 1

As the OT manager, you orient a new hire to the department and facility. After a three-month probationary period, you review the employee's performance. During that time minimal feedback was given to the staff person about being consistently late for appointments with consumers. Now you must decide whether or not to extend the probationary period, approve the employee for hire, or dismiss the employee.

Although timeliness with patients has been a problem, the staff person is very thorough and spends extra time with consumers. This individual makes effort to communicate to all team members about the progress of the consumer, and is well liked by them and all co-workers.

Discussion Questions

1. Write an employee goal sheet (using Figure 4.1) for initial planning at time of orientation. Use any area of practice in the field of occupational therapy.

2. Write an action plan to correct the area preventing maximum performance, in other words timeliness.

3. As the manager, what decision should be made regarding the employee's future in this position?

4. What should have been done differently in the first three months with this employee? Give examples.

5. Document the probationary meeting, including discussion of employee strengths, weaknesses, decisions made, and commitments agreed upon by both parties.

CHAPTER 5

Marketing the OT Program or Clinic

Marketing begins with a mission and develops into a useful tool through investigation and self-discovery. If correctly pursued, it is coordinated with the business plan to create a strategic marketing plan. Implemented successfully, a marketing program can promote growth and establish a presence in the community.

An independent practitioner, business owner, or department manager will need to be involved in marketing and self-promoting. Marketing one's profession and self is also imperative of the department therapists. Visibility creates awareness, and this will lead to referrals and contracts. A positive and honest portrayal of the services offered should characterize all marketing attempts. The consumer will trust and patronize a business with a solid, reputable image and values.

At the conclusion of this chapter, the reader will be able to:

1. Determine a marketing strategy appropriate to their department or clinic.

2. Choose types of marketing and advertising techniques to increase visibility within the community.

3. Be comfortable with marketing his- or herself and the profession of occupational therapy.

Strategizing the Market Plan

There are several steps in establishing a successful marketing program. Initially, a strengths, weaknesses, opportunities, and threats (SWOT) analysis is completed as discussed in Chapters 1 and 3. By identifying the strengths, weakness, opportunities, and threats of a department, a foundation is built for the strategic plan.

Secondly, determining how the department or clinic is different from its competitors is key. Hillestad and Berkowitz (1991) describe the differentiation strategy of marketing. It is used during the initial and growth stages of a program or practice. This method helps a program to gain advantage over a competitor by identifying the program strengths and learning from the competitor's weaknesses. The differential competitive advantage establishes how the consumer's needs are met by the program and lacking by the competition. Figures 5.1, 5.2, 5.3, and 5.4 can be used to identify the competitive advantage of a practice and strengthen its position in the market.

Answer the following questions with collaboration from OT staff.

1. What does your business offer that is unique to the community?

2. How do these services differ from the competition?

3. List all competitors.

4. What are the strengths of your competitors?

5. What are the weaknesses of the competition?

6. How can your business capitalize on competitor's weaknesses?

7. How can your business respond to the strengths of the competitors?

8. How can you business strengthen its market "niche"?

Figure 5.1. Finding a Market Niche

Complete the following information to identify the market for traditional and non-traditional OT services

1. Who are the consumers?

2. What are the needs of each consumer?

3. Are the needs of the consumer being met? If not, what are the areas of need?

4. What marketing approach is most appropriate for each consumer?

5. What are the settings presently served?

6. How can these services be improved?

7. What settings could be targeted for future services and why?

8. What marketing techniques will be used to address new or underserved populations?

Figure 5.2. Defining the Consumer

Complete the questions below when expanding services.

1. Who are your primary referral sources?

2. Why do they refer?

3. Are their needs being met?

4. How are they acknowledged for referrals given?

5. Who are your occasional referral sources?

6. Are their needs being met?

7. How can referrals be increased by these sources?

8. Who are the potential referral sources?

9. Why don't they refer?

10. What marketing approach is appropriate for occasional and potential referral sources?

Figure 5.3. Marketing to Expand Services

Develop a Market Plan for a more effective approach to consumers

Marketing goals:

1.

2.

3.

4.

5.

Marketing approach:	Date to be completed by:
1.	1.
2.	2.
3.	3.
4.	4.
5.	5.

Type of follow up to marketing:

1.

2.

3.

4.

5.

How will effectiveness be determined?

1.

2.

3.

4.

5.

Figure 5.4. Marketing Plan

A consumer evaluation and marketing strategy form is used to identify areas where additional referrals and programs may be established. The market segment analysis is used to review the consumer need for specific services and determine the possibility of new programs related to a market. Full understanding of the market position is achieved by becoming familiar with not only the program being promoted but all its competitors, as discussed in Chapter 3.

Another part of strategizing the market plan is to identify areas with growth potential and eliminate or decrease those services that are unprofitable and unlikely to grow. An OT manager may choose to promote only those services and programs that are strong and noteworthy.

In the early stages of a department or new program, however, public exposure to all available services is important. At this stage, bombarding the community and its consumers with as much information as possible is necessary to jump-start initial growth. This is done by frequent and repetitive advertising as instructed later in this chapter.

Following the planning stages of the market strategy, implementation of the promotion program begins. It is now necessary to determine the methods of advertisement, who will be targeted, when and where the marketing strategies will be used, and how often the promotions will be offered.

Why Advertise?

Many recommend use of a professional advertising or marketing agency to assist with the development of promotional materials. Although it is possible to implement marketing objectives without outside advice, it has been said that advertising is expensive when ineffective. (Bangs, 1998b)

When establishing the marketing objectives, the question "what is to be achieved by advertising?" must be answered. The purpose of the plan will alter decisions about what type of media is chosen. The answer for OT departments may be:

- Increase referrals
- Raise public awareness
- Maintain visibility
- Introduce services to the medical community
- Promote a new service

Methods of Promotions and Advertising

Paid advertising is a method of attempting to reach the public through multimedia. Numerous options exist and choices for this type of marketing should be customized to the purpose, budget, and schedule of the advertising campaign.

For example, a small department with low budget is interested in increasing awareness of fall prevention. A decision to run the ad in an insert targeted to senior citizens in the local newspaper was made. It will run for two consecutive weeks. A news release will be submitted in the same newspaper during subsequent weeks explaining fall prevention. The cost for this promotion is approximately $100 for both ads, including two news releases. Coverage is for one month at one time per week. It is important to note that in this plan, paid promotions are supplemented with news releases.

Paid endorsements include radio and TV commercials and newspaper advertising. More costly exposure from these media sources can offset cost by the significant number of viewers and listeners reached by this method. Experts recommend running these types of ads in consecutives blocks, e.g., ten times in a day or five times in a week, as opposed to one time per day for ten days, or one time per week for five weeks. By bombarding the market (submitting frequent and repetitious ads) even briefly, the ad is more likely to be remembered by its audience.

Radio

Paid advertising is used for short (usually thirty second) messages. Scripts are written by either the station, sales representative, marketing agency, or the individual submitting the ad. It can be read personally by the submitter, by a hired professional, or in some cases by an ad representative at the radio station. "Spots" are usually run multiple times during a day or week. Special promotions offered by the station can often make radio advertising affordable.

Public radio station advertising is also beneficial and is referred to as underwriting. A message is submitted and run at specific times designated by the purchaser of the ad. Choices about which programs are sponsored can be made as rates vary per days and times.

Public service announcements are *free* on public and private radio stations. They are beneficial to notify the public about free screenings, open houses, and OT month activities for example.

Television

Television ads can be run on network, cable, or satellite TV. Prices vary greatly by region and network. Reduction in cost can also be realized during non-peak hours and programs. Scripting and taping of TV commercials is performed jointly between the station and the OT department. This, of course, varies geographically, but in many areas, the OTs can even participate in the acting, editing, and choice of music. The final production is always approved by the OT administrator prior to completion. Because television ads are viewed by many consumers, this method of advertising is recommended if the budget allows.

Newspaper

News releases are *free* and should be utilized to promote OT and the services provided. The intent of a news release is to inform the public of information in the community. Therefore, the opening of a business or program, hiring of a new therapist, attendance at/or presenting of a workshop, scheduling of an open house, free screenings, or any educational topic of interest can be submitted.

Paid newspaper advertising varies in price based on size of ad, geographical location, day of week, and possibly placement of ad. Sales representatives are trained to assist the OT manager in creation of an appropriate ad. A hired marketing representative can also be helpful to prepare professional looking newspaper ads.

Back Door Promotion

In OT departments, business is often generated by physician or colleague referrals. In this scenario, it is assumed that others know and understand OT services and what benefits are received. If a practice is to depend solely on this method of obtaining referrals, little advertising budget will be required. However, full potential for referrals will probably not be realized in this case because many do *not* comprehend the realm of services occupational therapy can offer. Therefore, they need to be enlightened, and this is often the role of the OT manager. This can be done through:

- Newsletters
- Direct mailing
- Brochures
- News releases
- Personal contact
- Inservices
- Speaking engagements
- TV or radio interviews
- Regular news columns

Educating the public in this manner is also effective to elicit self-referrals. Many pharmaceutical companies obtain sales by prompting the consumer, through ads, to inquire about a medication with their physician. The same approach can be effective for OT. The consumer is given adequate information about their condition through news releases and advertising to request from their physician a referral for OT services. By sparking their attention to therapy as an option for their condition, the consumer becomes an advocate for himself or herself. In most situations, the referring source is willing to prescribe therapy when asked, especially if they are familiar in advance with the requested treatment.

World Wide Web

Internet advertising has become very popular and can serve to meet the goals of many OT businesses. When the market extends to state, national, or international levels, there is no question this media is imperative. An OT department sponsoring continuing education seminars will want to access the public in this way, for instance. There are many companies providing web page design and set-up, so the task can be less daunting for those OT managers wearing the hat of marketing director.

Yellow Pages

Often overlooked as part of the marketing plan is yellow page advertising. If a consumer is unable to find a telephone number to a business, they are likely to go elsewhere. Make it easy to find the services offered in an OT department with several listings in the directory. Check how the competitors utilize the telephone book, and attempt to overshadow them by using shaded or highlighted text, bold or multiple listings, same page ads, or colored ads. As stated previously, program names beginning with an early alphabetical listing may be chosen first in this type of media.

There are unlimited ways to spend money on promotions, therefore, it is prudent to be discriminating about the effectiveness of special directories and other forms of advertising. Community directories, church bulletins, ads on sports programs and grocery bags, telephone book cover ads, to name a few, may or may not provide the exposure a program is looking for.

Signage

Billboard presentations at sporting events, roadsides, sides of buildings, buses, or in subways are also options for paid promotions. Care should be taken, however, to create the desired image with the method of display. The type/location of service should be compatible with the location of the ad and its intended audience. For example, a softball field billboard would be more appropriate if promoting treatment of sports injuries than home health care.

In addition, a promotion needs to show a professional appearance. An OT clinic sign located in close proximity to only fast food restaurants and motel signs may be overlooked by potential consumers.

Health Fairs

Presence at local health fairs can boost community awareness of a program and its services. Offering an interactive-type booth (e.g., pediatric screenings) will spark interest for individuals to visit the booth. A good opportunity also exists here to distribute written flyers, information packets, business cards, and specialty items (personalized pens, "get a grip" jar openers, etc).

Open House

Inviting the public and medical/professional community in to an OT department is often a large undertaking, but worth the effort. The AOTA has promotional ideas for use at OT month events. There are many interactive techniques to involve the public while demonstrating the purpose of OT. For example, an ice cream social requiring use of adaptive equipment and props to prepare a sundae is a fun and engaging event. Carpal tunnel screenings can also draw interest to the open house.

Exploiting new building or remodeling, new staff, and anniversaries can also present opportunities for an open house. Open houses are most beneficial if they are well attended. Planning and publicity of these events will impact success. Door prizes, food, free screenings, educational materials, and convenient times increase the likelihood of good attendance. Posters, public service announcements, direct mailings, news releases, and possibly even TV news will increase awareness. Use every opportunity to capitalize on free visibility.

Every individual who enters the department once will be more likely to return for future visits if necessary. Make their first impression a positive one by portraying a friendly, caring, professional image. If a business is trusted, it will succeed.

Free Promotions

News releases, public service announcements (PSAs), direct letters, telephone calls, visits to physician offices, and presentations at service clubs, support groups, medical conferences, specialty groups, safety director group meetings, and employee staff meetings are all examples of "free" promotions. Some community newspapers would entertain a weekly or monthly column such as "rehab corner." Appendix 5.1 is an example of a type of consumer information column that could be offered on a continuous basis.

These types of promotions are used to solidify an OT's place in the community as an expert in an area of interest. They should be entered into cautiously, however, due to the time commitment involved in writing the ongoing segment.

Self-promotion

Telephone contact and personal letters constitute most attempts at self-promoting. Consider scheduling face-to-face visits at the individual's place of employment, a restaurant, or at the business being promoted. Offer to buy coffee or a meal. Make the meeting convenient for the individual, planning a block of time allowing to wait for them if necessary.

Be persistent and begin with the least threatening contact. Make a list of target individuals and meet with or contact them strategically. Do not give up until the list is exhausted. Every effort in this area will be rewarded with referrals and new professional relationships which can be very rewarding.

Some professional contacts to consider when self-promoting include:

- Physicians
- Physicians assistants
- Nurse practitioners
- RNs and rehabilitation nurses
- Case managers
- Discharge planners
- Social workers
- Teachers
- Safety directors
- Human resource directors
- School administrators
- Chiropractors
- Rehabilitation directors
- Other rehabilitation colleagues, i.e., physical and speech therapists
- School psychologists
- Insurance companies
- Politicians

Workshop Sponsorship

Offering local workshops and training sessions to target groups can increase visibility. Occupational therapists have a large body of knowledge and can offer many topics of interest to the community. Speaking engagements regarding ADA compliance, carpal tunnel syndrome prevention, back school, proper lifting techniques, stress management, fall prevention, and arthritis education are only a few of the areas to market to businesses, industry, support groups, etc.

Other

Membership in service clubs, volunteer efforts, and sponsorship of sports teams are obvious attempts to give back to the community. These acts are respected by many and can return their rewards to the organization in the form of personal gratification, as well as public awareness.

Involvement in OT professional organizations such as state and national associations can only serve to improve contacts, credibility, competence, and the knowledge to be an effective OT manager. In addition, networking in this way can increase contacts for future recruitment and referral potential. Active involvement in area OT school functions can produce good networking results and expand resources also.

Communicating Missions and Outcomes

In correspondence and promotions, personal contact, and education materials, identify the mission and intent of the service. In other words, verbalize to others that "our goal is to offer personalized service in a professional and caring atmosphere." Communicate any outcomes that have been collected and promote the benefits to the consumer; for example, "84% of carpal tunnel patients report prevention of surgery," "86% report that they are satisfied with the outcome of therapy." If any statistics have been compiled, make sure that referral sources, insurance companies, and the public are made aware.

Marketing Oneself

The ability to market one's skills is especially necessary when paving a road for occupational therapists in nontraditional settings. However, being able to sell oneself to others professionally is a great asset, which will elicit confidence from consumers, referral sources, potential employers, and colleagues.

Self-assurance in one's abilities to perform a task or competently learn a skill is fundamental to bring about an interest in what is being offered. Deficiencies in professional self-confidence must be addressed if successful self-marketing is to be realized. Some strategies to improve professional self-assurance are:

- Make a list of strengths and weaknesses.
- Seek opportunities which require skills in strength areas.
- Use self-affirmations.
- Write an action plan to address weaknesses.
- Practice expressing positive qualities (role playing).
- Identify how positive qualities benefit others.
- Identify why others may seek these qualities.
- Find a trusted mentor and seek constructive feedback.

When promoting oneself, be cognizant of the other party's interest and aware of their time constraints. Keep open communication flowing by keying into their primary agenda, if known. Anticipate their wants and needs and offer ways to address them. Remaining comfortable in an active listening mode will allow information to be collected while stimulating respect for the interest shown. Express how the skills possessed are compatible with their needs. Be honest about any lack of experience by openly expressing reservations you may have. If possible, provide solutions to these concerns, such as researching the skill, consulting with others, offering to be trained on a volunteer basis, etc. It is possible to lack knowledge in a specific area and still be of valuable service to others if one is motivated to learn.

When meeting with others in a marketing capacity, allow positive qualities and skills to be apparent so the other party can easily identify them. In other words, smile openly, be friendly and polite, listen actively, be honest, do not make others wonder about the interest and potential possessed, describe and give examples of previous experiences that are applicable to the needs that are being sought.

Marketing Occupational Therapy as a Profession

Many occupational therapists have difficulty explaining what OT is." This is the first step in being comfortable marketing the profession. Write a simple description and memorize it so that this question can be satisfied when *anyone* asks, from a potential employer to a relative, to the local hairdresser, or a business associate.

By focusing on the functional outcomes facilitated by occupational therapists, one can put the profession in "real life" terminology, which is understandable to most who are unfamiliar with OT. For example, occupational therapy addresses the "occupation" of an individual and strives to regain, or promote maximum function in daily life skills such as schoolwork, job skills, homemaking, bathing and dressing, or leisure activities.

Marketing tools exist to make this task easier and are available through the American Occupational Therapy Association and many state associations. Creating individualized marketing tools for a program or clinic, i.e., brochures and handouts, is highly appropriate, increases visibility, and substantiates OT as a profession within the community.

Documenting a Plan

Because marketing can be a long-term project, the use of measurable goals and timelines are no less important here than in a treatment plan. Set up a timeline to attack each promotion outlined in the advertising plan. Some recommend having a calendar with specific promotional plans, costs, and frequencies entered. This method can be used to schedule face-to-face contacts and even phone calls. Stay organized and structured, and follow through will be easier to assess and goals can be identified. Completion of a marketing budget can also be monitored in this manner.

Summary

Beginning with a mission statement and SWOT analysis, a department develops its market strategy. Self and competitive analyses are useful tools in determining the differentiation between products.

A timeline, budget, and promotional plan are tied to the advertising objectives of a department. Once a program understands what its purpose of advertising is, plans can be made to implement the strategy developed to increase awareness, visibility, and understanding of the OT services offered. Successful completion of this plan will stimulate referrals, contracts, employees, and business.

Case Study 1

An occupational therapist has a casual social encounter with a new business owner. Fifty individuals are employed there and in the first year, two cases of carpal tunnel syndrome have been claimed. The new employer is very interested your occupation and requests additional information about what OTs can offer.

Discussion Questions

1. What is the response of the OT?
2. Is it ethical to discuss this at a social gathering?
3. What materials, if any, should be supplied to the business owner?
4. What does OT have to offer this employer and the employees?
5. Who is the consumer?

Case Study 2

A busy neurology clinic that provides consistent referrals to an OT department hired a new physician. What should the OT department do?

Project #1

Write an article for a weekly medical section of the local paper. Promote OT through public information aimed at a group of individuals with a specific health need.

Project #2

Create an ad to be published in a newspaper or one to be recorded for radio. The purpose of the ad is to inform the community about the OT services provided. Design a fictitious program for the ad.

CHAPTER 6

Documentation

Effective written communication is required of the occupational therapist. Documentation is used to describe the occupational therapy treatment program, goals, outcomes, and recommendations. It is a method of justifying continuation of the treatment program or discharge from occupational therapy services. Documentation is an integral part of communication to the referring source, caregiver, case manager, third party payer, and team members and is a legal record of the consumer's occupational therapy status. Reimbursement is often dependent upon complete documentation.

At the conclusion of this chapter, the reader will be able to:

1. Understand the types and content of occupational therapy reports.

2. Understand documentation requirements.

3. Know the documentation elements necessary for reimbursement.

Content of the Medical Record

There are elements of the medical record that, if absent, may prompt payment denial upon review by many fiscal intermediaries. They include:

- Physician referral and re-certification every 30 days;
- Patient medical history, provided by patient or a physician
- Initial evaluation findings and present functional status
- Long and short term goals
- Daily treatment notes
- Monthly or weekly progress notes including outcomes of goal attainment.

The AOTA has established guidelines for occupational therapy record keeping in "Elements of Clinical Documentation" found in Appendix 6.1. Although practice settings may alter the type of documentation required, these guidelines will assist the OT manager in establishing a complete and competent clinical record keeping system that may help to assure reimbursement for services provided and thorough written communication with the referring source.

In addition, the descriptors used to report OT services must contain that which has already been established by the AOTA in "Uniform Terminology for Occupational Therapy—Third Edition. This document is found in Appendix 6.2.

Report Style

Documentation format may change based on the type of report. The style can be individualized to person, facility, or practice setting but the primary categories and content areas should remain the same regardless of the format used. Narrative and SOAP (subjective, objective, assessment, plan) styles are both widely accepted. Figure 6.1 shows an example of a SOAP note and Figure 6.2 gives an example of a narrative report format. The practitioner should always keep in mind that the purpose of the report is to communicate to others, i.e., referral source, funding source, etc.

Consumer functional status and documentation of service provided by the therapist are content areas that should never be omitted from report writing. Therapists should be encouraged to be clear and concise, while keeping the reader in mind. The reader must be able to interpret the meaning and intent of the report.

Reimbursement Consideration

Because documentation is the primary method of communication, this is also what determines payment if a question exists regarding frequency, duration, or medical necessity of treatment. The following areas are targeted during a medical record review.

Physician Referral

The prescription for occupational therapy from the physician should contain several elements: consumer name and treatment diagnosis, date of referral, type of evaluation and treatment requested, and date of onset of the treating diagnosis. Estimated length of treatment required to facilitate change in functional improvement should also be included. Verbal orders may be received if followed by a written referral.

Physician Certification of the Therapy Program

Having physician signatures on treatment plans is required for recertification of occupational therapy services a minimum of every thirty days for some third party payers including Medicare. A stamped signature is not accepted for recertification and date must be on or before the thirtieth day from the start of initial evaluation or first date of treatment. For consumers requiring ongoing therapy, this process is repeated each month. In addition, the physician must see the patient every thirty days to determine continued need for occupational therapy services, and should also document an anticipated length of time required to meet the therapy goals. Reimbursement for Medicare services is dependent upon compliance in this area.

Functional Reporting and Goal Writing

For purposes of assuring that documentation leads to reimbursement, it is important to identify some common errors in documentation. One common problem in documentation is poorly written goals that do not address functional performance and are not measurable. A goal to "improve trunk control"

OCCUPATIONAL THERAPY DISCHARGE SUMMARY

PT. NAME: **PHYSICIAN:**

DOB: **DATE OF REPORT:**

PHONE: **DATE OF ONSET:**

ADDRESS: **DIAGNOSIS:**

SUBJECTIVE:

Patient feels that she has good use of her L hand and reports that she is very aware of keeping her fingers in proper alignment when she is performing ADL. She also takes note to adjust the position of her fingers when resting her hand on a table or chair, etc.

_____ also, states that she now is able to do dishes, sweep the floor, and shovel snow (using her forearm to hold the shovel). Patient reports use of new adaptive equipment for meal preparation. She states that her L hand is feeling better every day. She continues to wear her splint at night for positioning purposes.

OBJECTIVE:

Patient was seen 2–3x/week for the first 4 weeks, then 1–2x/week for the next three weeks, weaning to 1x per week upon d/c. Sessions where initially 1 hour, decreasing to 30 min by the 6th week. Pt was seen in the clinic for a total of 16 visits.

Program implementation included design and fabrication of dynamic outrigger splint. Continued treatment was to monitor and adjust alignment of dynamic outrigger splint, instruct and monitor HEP for ROM of L digits. HEP was demonstrated for compliance.

Assistive devices for prevention were reviewed and patient was referred to appropriate vendor for adaptive equipment such as built up utensils. Functional activities were discussed and problem solving with family and patient occurred to maximize independence. It was determined that spouse will assist more for vacuuming and patient will utilize stool and wheeled cart in the kitchen during meal preparation.

Reevaluation measurements were obtained on this date and are as follows (01/04/99):

RANGE OF MOTION

L DIGITS	(INITIAL)		DISCHARGE	
(INDEX)	(AROM /	PROM)	(AROM /	PROM)
MP	15-56°	0-59°	0-60°	0-70°
PIP	23-85°	0-95°	0-105°	WNL
DIP	0-45°	0-55°	0-61°	0-70°
(LONG)	(AROM /	PROM)	(AROM /	PROM)
MP	35-60°	0-70°	10-70°	0-82°
PIP	21-84°	0-90°	0-108°	WNL
DIP	0-40°	0-45°	0-65°	0-68°
(RING)	(AROM /	PROM)	(AROM /	PROM)
MP	20-56°	0-65°	0-60°	0-71°
PIP	18-70°	7-75°	5-95°	WNL
DIP	0-12°	0-40°	0-30°	0-67°

Figure 6.1. Discharge (SOAP) Note for Outpatient (*continues*)

(SMALL)	INITIAL (AROM / PROM)		DISCHARGE (AROM / PROM)	
MP	0-31°	0-55°	0-45°	0-60°
PIP	30-72°	0-75°	20-100°	WNL
DIP	0-36°	0-45°	0-60°	0-67°

HEP was reassessed, and pt.'s spouse was present to help reinforce performance as well as compliance. Discussion regarding further surgeries for L thumb fusion indicated that pt. will continue with next surgery in approximately one month, which will be discussed with physician.

ASSESSMENT:

Although joint stiffness was noted on this reevaluation date, it appears that pt. has resumed good functional use of her L hand, and she is satisfied with the outcome of her surgery and therapy. Continued spontaneous progress is expected following discharge.

Patient is appropriate for discharge at this time, with the following goals being met as stated below:

LTG: Pt. will return to full functional use of her L hand for dressing, bathing, and homemaking, by 01/31/99. (GOAL MET)

STG 1: Pt. will be able to use L hand for dressing skills, manipulating buttons and other closures, by 12-1-98. (GOAL MET)

STG 2: Pt. will demonstrate ability to perform grooming and feeding tasks independently, by 12/15/98. (GOAL MET)

STG 3: Pt. will demonstrate AROM in L digits to within functional limits, by 12/31/98. (GOAL MET)

STG 4: Pt. will be able to prepare a light meal such as soup and sandwich or breakfast independently, by 1/15/99. (GOAL MET)

PLAN:

Will discharge pt. to physician's care with further follow-up provided p.r.n.

THANK YOU FOR THIS REFERRAL

_____
THERAPIST'S SIGNATURE

_____
PHYSICIAN'S SIGNATURE

_____
DATE

_____
DATE

Figure 6.1. Discharge (SOAP) Note for Medicare Outpatient *(continued)*

OCCUPATIONAL THERAPY
Initial Evaluation Summary

PT. NAME: **PHYSICIAN:**
DOB: **DATE OF REPORT:**

PHONE: **DATE OF ONSET:**
ADDRESS: **DIAGNOSIS:**

History

Present functional status

Evaluation findings
      ADLs

      Motor

      Sensory

      Cognitive

      Emotional

Rehab potential

Treatment plan

Interventions discussed and implemented

Recommendations/Plan

Figure 6.2. Narrative Format for Documentation

falls into this category, but could be changed easily to address function. "The patient will demonstrate necessary trunk control to independently bathe self while seated on a tub bench, within thirty days" is another way of stating the same goal in terms specific to a patient's independent status, with a measurable outcome.

Occupational therapists can continue to strengthen their roles in the rehabilitation process by communicating the extent to which consumers are brought to greater independence and function. The role of occupational therapy in prevention and wellness can also be expanded in the same way. Outcomes from therapy should not be in terms of range of motion, strength, endurance, sensation, behaviors, or cognition unless they are directly related to what functional gains were noted as a result.

In other words, how does a decrease in tactile defensiveness improve a child's ability to function? Why does a carpenter need a goal to increase grip strength? How does someone benefit from the ability to use his or her dominant hand? Why will building self-esteem be important to a depressed individual interested in obtaining a job? How can increasing attention span improve independence in a homemaker, student, or worker? If pain interferes in the ability to sleep, how does this impair function? How will training foster parents of special needs children promote function within the family? If these types of questions are answered when documenting progress, the purpose of OT will be maintained and the reader will clearly understand the intent of intervention.

A "5-ingredient recipe" for functional goal writing may be:

KEY **PLAYER**

+

FUNCTIONAL **PERFORMANCE**

+

THE **CHANGE** EXPECTED

+

AMOUNT OF CHANGE EXPECTED

+

WHEN EXPECTED

=

MEASURABLE FUNCTIONAL GOAL

Establishing measurable goals with patient input will increase the consumer's interest in the treatment program as well as strengthen report writing skills necessary for medical review standards.

Medicare Documentation Review

Review of the medical records by the Medicare intermediary is performed methodically or on a random basis based on payer preference at any given time. Reviews are done in two classifications: Level I Review and Level II Review. Although an overview is provided below, detailed information regarding Medicare documentation and reimbursement guidelines is found in one of the many Medicare publications. These government documents, specific to areas of practice and setting, provide all necessary information for completing correct documentation, thereby maximizing reimbursement.

Among those manuals of interest to the OT manager are:

- *Medicare Outpatient Physical Therapy and Comprehensive Outpatient Rehabilitation Facility Manual*

  HCFA Pub. 9, PB 98-950100

- *Medicare Hospital Manual*

  HCFA Pub. 10, PB 98-955100

- *Medicare Home Health Agency Manual*

  HCFA Pub. 11, PB 98-955200

- *Medicare Skilled Nursing Facility Manual*

  HCFA Pub. 12, PB 98-954900

The above publications are available at the HCFA website in the publications section. These manuals are facility complete, therefore, extremely lengthy. It is suggested that they be reviewed for information specific to OT before they are downloaded.

The Medicare *Program Integrity Manual* is the first Internet only manual and contains information for the OT administrator in outpatient services. It includes DME and other pertinent policy information and can be seen in its entirety at www.hcfa.gov/pubforms/83%5Fpim/pim83c06.htm.

A section of this manual, "Guidelines for Special Services," Ch. 6, Sec. 7, is specific to occupational therapy and can be downloaded on the Internet by going to Chapter 6, Section 7 at the above web address.

Components of the material regarding medical review (MR) and documentation are outlined below, with permission from the Health Care Financing Administration.

Level I Review

The use of occupational therapy edits has been developed for a number of diagnoses. Edits are guidelines for a predetermined number of therapy visits and total weeks seen per diagnosis prior to automatic record review. When linked to a recent onset date, the diagnosis indicates a probability that the Medicare consumer would require skilled occupational therapy. As described later in this chapter, compatibility of CPT and ICD-9 codes is also necessary. Complete documentation is paramount because if claims pass the Level I edit process, a Level II medical review is not necessary.

The information being reviewed at Level I is based upon: 1) facility name, patient name, facility provider number, patient age; 2) primary diagnosis (ICD-9 CM Code) for which OT services were provided; 3) total duration of OT services (in days), 4) date of initial treatment, 5) billing.

Level II Review

If a claim is reviewed using the Level I criteria and is found to be questionable or inconsistent in terms of number of treatment days per diagnosis, types of treatment performed per diagnosis, etc., a Level II Review will be requested. When a Level II process is selected for medical review, additional medical information and documentation is requested of the provider.

The types of information being assessed at this level are:

- History which pertains to the treatment provided, brief description of the functional status of the consumer prior to the onset, and any prior occupational therapy services

- Date of onset—date on which primary medical diagnosis occurred for which services are being rendered

- Physician referral and date
- OT initial evaluation end date
- Plan of treatment and date established
- Date of last certification by physician
- Progress reports—updated patient status concerning consumer's current functional abilities and limitations.

Specific Level II Documentation Requirements

Medical History. The history of treatments from a previous provider is necessary for patients who have transferred to a new provider for the current condition. If the consumer has had prior therapy for the same condition, use that history in conjunction with the patient's current assessment to establish whether additional treatment is reasonable.

Evaluation. The provider documents the consumer's functional loss and the level of assistance requiring—*skilled* OT intervention resulting from conditions such as:

- Activities of daily living (ADL) dependence—Skilled intervention is performed due to significant physical and/or cognitive functional loss or loss of previous functional gains. This could include management and care of orthosis and/or adaptive equipment, or customized therapeutic adaptations.

- Functional limitation—Skilled OT intervention is required for functional training, observation, assessment, and environmental adaptation possibly due to lack of sensory awareness, safety hazards, impaired attention span, decreased strength, uncoordination, abnormal muscle tone, limitations in range of motion, impaired body scheme, impaired perception, impaired balance and head control, and environmental barriers.

- Safety dependence secondary to complications—This category implies that without skilled occupational therapy services, a consumer cannot handle him or herself in a manner that is physically and/or cognitively safe. This may extend to daily living or to acquired secondary complications which could potentially intensify medical sequelae, such as nonunion of a fracture or skin breakdown. Safety dependence may be demonstrated by a high probability of falling, lack of environmental safety awareness, inability to recognize danger, abnormal aggressive or destructive behavior, severe pain, loss of skin sensation, progressive joint contracture, joint protection and preservation, and swallowing difficulties requiring skilled OT intervention to protect the patient from further medical complication(s).

Plan of Treatment. This document includes specific functional goals and a reasonable estimate of when they will be reached (e.g., six weeks). It is not adequate to estimate "one to two months on an ongoing basis." The provider submits changes in the plan with the progress notes. The plan must include:

- Type of OT procedures.
- Frequency of visits—Estimate the frequency of expected treatment (e.g., three times per week). Medical documentation should justify the intensity of services expected, especially when provided greater than three times a week.

- Estimated duration—This documents the expected length of time treatment will be provided in days, weeks, or months.

- Diagnoses—Include the occupational therapy diagnosis, especially if different from the medical diagnosis. The OT diagnosis is based on objective tests, when appropriate, such as weakness, lack of motion, decreased functional ability, and sensory loss.

- Functional OT goals (short or long term)—Describe the functional physical/cognitive abilities the patient is expected to receive as established by therapist, consumer/family, and physician.

- Rehabilitation potential—Document the expectation concerning the patient's ability to meet the established goals. If the rehabilitation potential is not good, the individual should not be receiving skilled rehabilitation services.

Progress Reports. In addition to what was described about progress reports previously in this chapter, Medicare states that the progress report, otherwise referred to as a status summary, must document a continued expectation that the consumer's condition will continue to improve significantly in a reasonable and generally predictable period of time. "Significant" means a generally measurable and substantial increase in the patient's present level of functional independence and competence, compared to that when treatment was initiated. If a consumer experiences a medical complication for a brief period where a lack of progress occurs, therapy is considered reasonable if it can be documented that there is still an expectation that significant improvement in the patient's overall safety or functional ability will occur. The provider, therefore, should document the temporary lack of progress and justify the need for continued skilled OT.

If a consumer's full or partial recovery is not possible, i.e., if a terminally ill patient begins to exhibit ADL, mobility, and/or safety dependence requiring OT, the reviewer will look at documentation regarding whether the services are considered reasonable and effective treatment of the patient's condition and whether they require the skills of an occupational therapist. The reasons for OT must be clear, as well as its goals, prior to approval for coverage.

Intermediate gradations of improvement based on changes and behavior in response to assistance are found within the assistance levels of minimum, moderate, and maximum. Improvements at each level must be documented, comparing the current cognitive and/or physical levels achieved to previous function.

The consistent use of the terminology below, which describe objective performance measures, will clarify documentation and maximize reimbursement.

The following are standards for levels of assistance used for objective reporting of functional tasks as indicated in the Medicare Program Integrity Manual (HCFA 2000a). This information can be obtained at www.hcfa.gov/.

1. Total assistance—need for 100% assistance by one or more persons to perform all physical activities and/or cognitive assistance to elicit a functional response to an external stimulation.

2. Maximum assistance—the need for 75% assistance by one person to physically perform any part of a functional activity and/or cognitive assistance to perform gross motor actions in response to direction.

3. Moderate assistance—the need for 50% assistance by one person to perform physical activities or constant cognitive assistance to sustain/complete simple, repetitive activities safely.

4. Minimum assistance—need for 25% assistance by one person for physical activities under periodic, cognitive assistance to perform functional activities safely.

5. Stand-by assistance—the need for supervision by one person for the patient to perform new procedure adapted by the therapist for safe and effective performance.

6. Independent status—no physical or cognitive assistance is required to perform functional activities.

The following describes refusals, inconsistency and generalization as methods for reporting change:

1. Refusals—the patient may respond by refusing to attempt an activity because of fear or pain. Documentation should indicate the activity refused, the reasons, and how the OT plan addresses them.

2. Inconsistency—the patient may respond by inconsistently performing functional tasks from day to day or within a treatment session. The documentation must indicate a significant progress in consistency of performance of functional tasks within the same level of assistance.

3. Generalization—the patient may respond by applying previously learned concepts for performing an activity to another similar activity. To justify the occupational therapy services rendered, provide documentation of the scope and type of activities the patient can perform.

Medical Necessity

Requirements for medical necessity have become a significant issue for reimbursement by fiscal intermediaries including Medicare and Medicaid. For occupational therapy to be considered medically necessary, the services rendered must be those which only qualified occupational therapy personnel can perform. In other words, the skills and knowledge of an occupational therapist must be required for the consumer to make the expected functional gains. If a home program or caregiver could accomplish the task, the skilled occupational therapy services are not deemed to be medically necessary.

If spontaneous improvement in function is likely, or if the consumer makes no gains toward the established goals, treatment is also considered to lack medical necessity. Improvement must be interpreted to be significant, i.e., an increase in function is documented. The patient must have at least a fifty percent possibility of meeting the goals in a predicted period of time, based on the educated expectations and frequency and duration of therapy and considering diagnostic severity and prognosis of consumer.

"Determining if treatment is reasonable and necessary is also a method of granting reimbursement for occupational therapy services. Good or fair rehabilitation potential exists when the consumer is expected to improve significantly in a reasonable period of time on the basis of the occupational therapist's initial assessment." (HCFA, 2000b) Necessity of services can be argued when the special qualifications of an occupational therapist are required to bring the consumer to maximum functional potential. The treatment diagnosis, which may differ from the medical diagnosis, must be compatible with the services rendered in order to qualify for reasonable and necessary treatment.

Edits and Compatible Coding

Other necessities include documentation of appropriate diagnosis codes (ICD-9-CM) as they relate to specific procedure codes (Current Procedural Terminology-CPT) and any edits that exist. Edits refer to the designated visit and duration allowance prior to medical reviews for certain diagnoses. Edits and incompatible diagnosis codes will impact coverage of services. In other words, an example of an incompatible procedure diagnosis code mix would be a sensory integration procedure code for a consumer with a wrist fracture. A consumer with rheumatoid arthritis who received therapy for joint replacements will spark medical review if seen for 20 visits in 45 weeks.

Edit can be found in the Medicare procedure manual specific to area of practice and in the Program Integrity Manual for OPs in the enclosed CD-ROM.

ICD-9 codes are also located in the Medicare procedure manual, associated with the edits section. Complete ICD-9 listings can be reviewed at www.mcis.duke.edu/standards/termcare/icd-9/1tabular.html. In addition, there are certain CPT codes that when used simultaneously will be denied reimbursement and may prompt a MR.

Medicaid

Although Medicaid (MA) programs are administered by the Health Care Financing Administration (HCFA), each state has its own set of requirements and guidelines for participation in the program. Because OT is *not* one of the federally mandated benefits within the Medicaid program, it is incumbent upon the OT manager to determine the provision of OT coverage in the specific state. The reader is directed to the HCFA website at www.hcfa.gov/ for specific information for the state in which services will be provided.

Prior Authorization

Often MA administration programs recommend or require use of prior authorization requests (PAs) before OT services are implemented, after a preestablished number of visits for therapy services have been received in a lifetime, and/or for co-treatment situations. Documentation for PAs must include information about the extent of therapy, i.e., time/day, sessions/week, and projected duration. A description of the consumer's diagnosis, date of onset and associated problems, therapy history and brief pertinent history, evaluations used and results obtained, functional progress since last authorization, plan of care, and rehabilitation potential are requested by many states.

During implementation of the plan of treatment, MA requires a written entry for each date a consumer receives OT. The medical record must also contain the date and duration of treatment, problems treated, interventions and procedure codes, as well as objective measurement of consumer response to treatment.

Educational Settings

Public school districts have the same expectations for the content of therapy reports, but usually presented in a different format. Requirements are for annual Individual Educational Plan (IEP) goals developed with the team, evaluation report and three-year reevaluation report, and quarterly and annual summaries. Daily notes are optional in some school districts but recommended for accountability. A team representative completes the IEP review, revision, and placement documents as well as conducts the evaluation team meeting, with accompanying paperwork.

Some states have eliminated the need for physician referral for students continuing to receive OT in the educational model. This trend is expected to continue to more states in the future.

For forms used in the educational model, contact the local school district, or appropriate governing agency such as the state education department or department of public instruction.

Peer Review

A measure of accountability for quality and completeness of documentation as well as treatment decisions can be implemented with peer review policies. A checklist for assuring that all necessary documentation is intact will expedite the review process. Random review of several complete consumer records should be done each month by other staff. Reviewers are kept confidential to eliminate possible conflicts of interest.

Critical pathways or standards of care may be used to monitor quality of treatment through peer review. This process refers to the system of review in predetermined strategies (or pathways) that have been found to be effective for treating specific diagnostic groups or problem areas. For example, an individual who had hip replacement surgery should have documented evidence of receiving the following minimum of treatments from OT beginning on the second day of admission and completed prior to discharge from inpatient hospitalization: instruction of proper hip precautions during activities of daily living and demonstration with use of adaptive equipment for dressing and bathing.

Therapy files are scrutinized for appropriateness of the treatment program, success of goal achievement, and length of treatment. The purpose of implementing a therapy peer review program is to insure appropriate quality and quantity of services. A peer review form such as that seen in Figure 6.3 can be used to assess completeness of documentation.

Accreditation agencies such as Joint Commission on Accreditation of Healthcare Organizations (JCAHO) and Commission on Accreditation of Rehabilitation Facilities (CARF) require presence of such quality improvement programs. To be successful, this type of program must have follow-up with an action plan for correcting any deficiencies found.

Other Rules of Thumb for Clinical Record Keeping

A consumer file presents a complete picture of the rehabilitation process if maintained properly. The following list of guidelines is appropriate for traditional and nontraditional occupational therapy settings, including but not limited to the medical record:

- Be clear, concise and accurate.
- Avoid opinions.
- Never include judgments.
- Use black ink.
- Be legible.

PEER REVIEW
DOCUMENTATION AUDIT

Date of audit:

Chart reviewed:

Password of reviewer:

Therapist reviewed:

DOCUMENTATION CHECKLIST:	PRESENT IN CHART:	NOT PRESENT:
Physician order prior to tx initiation, including: Physician signature		
Recertification signature at least every 30 days		
Pertinent Medical Hx		
Prior level of function		
Present level of function (for progress and d/c reports)		
Objective findings		
Objective and subjective changes for progress and d/c reports		
Functional deficits		
Functional gains (for progress and d/c reports)		
Short-term goals are measurable, functional, and lead to long term goals		
Long term goals are measurable and functional		
Rehab potential is addressed		
Home exercise program is described		
Discussion with family, caregivers, and or team members is documented		
Daily note is present for each session billed		
Entry is complete for each procedure billed		
Progress is reported a minimum of every 30 days		
Consumer response to treatment indicated		
Diagnosis is compatible with procedures and length of treatment		

Figure 6.3. Peer Review Form *(continues)*

DOCUMENTATION CHECKLIST:	PRESENT IN CHART:	NOT PRESENT:
Medical necessity is evidenced by:		
Frequency of tx sessions (x's/week)		
Duration of tx (minutes/tx)		
Length of tx (weeks/months)		
Reason for d/c		
Recommendations		
Future		
Instruction to pt/caregiver		

STRENGTHS OF DOCUMENTATION

1.

2.

3.

4.

ACTION PLAN FOR OMISSIONS and DEFICIENCIES

Documentation omission or error: Plan to correct deficiency:

1.

2.

3.

4.

Figure 6.3. Peer Review Form *(continued)*

- Include only relevant content.
- Use "this therapist" or "this writer" when referring to self.

Forms and Computer Documentation

There are many situations where documentation is completed by standard forms required of the facility, fiscal intermediary, or government agency. Often they are completed with computer generation. Computerized programs for evaluation and documentation are becoming more prevalent with advances in technology. If used, some offer the ability to collect outcomes data, generate reports, and objectively communicate information about the consumer.

Medicare 700 and 701 Forms

Some states, fiscal intermediaries, and facilities mandate use of the HCFA 700/701 forms for documentation of OT services provided to Medicare recipients. In all cases, the information requested in the 700/701 must be included in the documentation for each Medicare recipient, if these forms are not used. Complete documentation information can be obtained for the HCFA 700 in Appendix A-7.3 and for the 701 Form in Appendix A-7.4, which can be downloaded free of charge at www.hcfa.gov/pubforms/. Any question whether the forms are current should be resolved by contacting HCFA or the appropriate HCFA contractor.

Minimal Data Set (MDS) 2.0

This computer generated resident assessment instrument is nationally mandated for use in collecting and recording resident data in skilled nursing facilities (SNFs). Historically, this was used as a nursing tool in long term care settings. The MDS is a primary driving force in reimbursement levels and a target for state inspections. It includes minutes of therapy time implemented and is used to establish a resident utilization group (RUG) category, which then determines the amount of reimbursement eligibility. Information for use of this document can also be obtained from the Health Care Financing Administration at www.hcfa.gov/medicaid/mds20/default.htm.

Medicare OASIS

This tool is used for documentation of home health care services. It is a software-based system that collects outcomes for home health care recipients for use by providers. According to HCFA, it is designed to represent core items of a comprehensive assessment for adult home care consumers, and forms a basis for measuring outcomes for purposes of outcome based quality improvement (OBQI). Data entry is completed with the HAVEN data entry system. Information for this tool can be obtained at www.hcfa.gov/medicare/hsqb/oasis/104.staff.htm.

OT Fact

Documentation programs such as OT FACT (www.execpc.com/~dgtldesn.otfact.htm) have been developed for ease in record keeping and outcome measurement. This functional performance evaluation is a data collection system that allows the therapist to compare the consumer functional status at initial, interim, and discharge evaluations. Systems such as OT FACT enable the therapist to have documented outcomes to substantiate decisions to continue or discontinue treatment.

Functional Independence Measure (FIM)

The FIM is a widely used evaluation tool that allows the therapist to objectively monitor outcomes about consumer functional status. This measurement device provides a source of data to supplement the requirements of thorough documentation. Further information can be obtained at www.neuro.wustl.edu/stroke-scales/fim.htm and will be addressed again in Chapter 8 for use in outcomes measurement.

Summary

The importance of adequate written communication cannot be underestimated. Reimbursement, coordination of care, and communication of relevant findings and work performed are among the reasons to place high priority on written communication. Complete record keeping provides a legal description of services rendered. Any discrepancies brought forth are always checked against the information recorded for dates of service in question. Incomplete or inaccurate documentation can have devastating results if put to the test through medical review or the court process. It is very important to note that billing for services which are not supported by proper documentation is considered fraudulent and can be prosecuted by the state and federal government.

Although documentation can be daunting for some therapists, it is the responsibility of each individual provider and the OT manager to assure proper record keeping. Peer review can benefit therapists with poor documentation skills. The time spent at this task can be alleviated somewhat with computerized reporting, dictation, flow sheets, and good organizational skills. Advancing technologies are expected to increase ease and speed in the record keeping process.

Case Study

Complete a peer review of the document in Figure 6.1 using the Peer Review Documentation Audit (Figure 6.3). Answer the questions below to determine thoroughness of report writing for this consumer.

Discussion Questions

1. Are all the elements of clinical documentation found in this report? If not, what would you have the therapist include?
2. If you were a medical claims reviewer, what additional records would you request to determine medical necessity?
3. What progress has the consumer made toward the treatment goals, if any?
4. Do you feel this claim should be paid with the information you were provided?

CHAPTER 7

Reimbursement

Reimbursement policy and billing procedures are at the core of all changes and regulations in payment systems. Occupational therapy services have been impacted by these changes in the form of reimbursement rates and payer policy resulting in reductions of coverage allowed. In moving from a fee for service system which paid for actual services billed on an individual basis, to a prospective payment system (PPS) with reimbursement based on average cost for a specific diagnosis or diagnostic related group (DRG), the frequency and duration of OT visits have been drastically impacted. Therapists have learned to prioritize treatments and maximize effectiveness, while attaining positive outcomes in shorter periods of time, in order for payment to be authorized and department profits to be realized.

At the conclusion of this chapter, the reader will be able to:

1. Understand the methods for submitting claims for OT services to fiscal intermediaries and insurance carriers.

2. Implement the use of the universal coding systems for diagnosis and procedures.

3. Know how to contact state insurance commissioners to obtain local guidelines.

4. Understand the channels required to receive pre- or prior authorization before treatment begins.

5. Know where to go to find details about reimbursement procedures and guidelines for government funded insurance programs.

6. Become aware of billing forms needed for claims submission.

Managed Care

Presently, preferred provider organizations (PPOs) and health maintenance organizations (HMOs) operate in a managed care system. The payer approves chosen providers to be a part of their organization, and to deliver health care services with arrangements to accept a predetermined fee, discounted rate, or capitated rate for their treatment. Capitation rates allow a fixed reimbursement rate per recipient in the plan over a determined period of time for all services provided during that specified period of time. The OT manager negotiating the capitation rate must carefully predict the number of enrollees who might require care. In addition, the type of care and length of treatment must be considered and calculated if a profit is to be realized in a capitation payment system.

In today's scenario, the payer is the gatekeeper of care for the consumer. Although some PPOs require the consumer or "member" to choose from a fixed provider group, others give financial incentives for choosing those within the specified group of providers. If the consumer receives treatment outside of the provider group, additional rates apply, usually in the form of percent of charges or a high deductible; for example, 80 percent coverage within the plan, 60 percent coverage for out of plan services, or $5,000 deductible for nonparticipating providers.

For an independent practitioner or business, or an existing department or group to be accepted as participating providers, an application process must be completed. Usually the carrier's provider relations or contracting department is responsible for this process and should be contacted initially via telephone. They can inform the applicant of the appropriate procedure and will mail an application. Professional references are required at times, and always a copy of each provider's diploma and certification must be submitted.

Some HMOs and PPOs will deny entry to the provider or group for a variety of reasons, such as closed enrollment or enough persons in a discipline and geographical area available. Therefore, it may be helpful to supply consumer letters of support, justification of outcomes, and most importantly evidence of cost savings for the carrier with the application. (If, for example, a provider can document that due to patient satisfaction with treatment, 25 people in one year have opted not to have surgery for carpal tunnel syndrome, the carrier may be more interested in using that provider's services.) Frequent and repetitive application may be necessary before provider status is confirmed.

Medicare

Medicare provides health insurance benefits for individuals over 65 years of age, those with permanent kidney failure, and some disabled persons. The government funds the program from payroll taxes and has set up fiscal intermediaries in various regions of the country to manage the Medicare systems in each region.

Therapists interested in becoming independent providers for the Medicare program must complete the enrollment procedure for the state of interest. To determine the appropriate managing intermediary, see Appendix A-7.1, Medicare Fiscal Intermediaries by State. Downloading the enrollment application from the Internet or calling the customer service department for the intermediary and requesting an application through the mail can begin the enrollment process.

Occupational therapy providers are considered non-physician providers. Download the application from www.noridian.com/medweb. Click on the state of interest, then on the provider enrollment prompt. Filing of the applications when received may take 30 to 45 days minimum, but some intermediaries allow a retroactive effective date, if needed for patient care and billing.

For services to be considered a covered procedure under Medicare guidelines, they must be referred by a physician, performed by a qualified occupational therapist or qualified occupational therapy assistant with appropriate supervision (as determined by Medicare), and be considered reasonable and necessary for the treatment of the individual's illness or injury.

Regulations for Medicare change frequently and are submitted to the provider on a monthly basis, in the form of a newsletter called the *Communique*. Updated information is also available at the Heath Care Financing Administration (HCFA) website at www.hcfa.gov/.

Medicare intermediary manuals define the rules established under the Medicare program manuals and forms can be downloaded or ordered through the website: www.hcfa.gov/pubforms/default.htm, also mentioned in Chapter 6, Documentation. Much of the information of interest to OT managers is found in the *Program Integrity Manual,* Pub 83, Chapter 6: Intermediary Guidelines for Specific Services, however all sites and areas of practice are covered in manuals from this website.

The Balanced Budget Act (BBA) of 1997, P.L.105-33, caused implementation of changes in Medicare reimbursement that continue to be challenged and revised today. Recently the BBA Refinement Act (BBRA) of 1999 put a two-year moratorium on an outpatient cap of $1500 for OT claims with services dated 1-1-2000 through 12-31-01. Although these claims will not be subject to this financial limitation, they may be reviewed to ensure reasonable and necessary services were rendered. These changes which have been in effect in SNFs since 1998 can be expected to affect inpatient rehabilitation beginning in April 2001.

The present system pays providers using a per diem PPS for SNFs covering *all* costs (routine, ancillary, and capital) related to the services furnished to beneficiaries under Part A of the Medicare program, (HCFA 2000b). HCFA also describes the per diem payments for each admission as case-mix adjustment: using a resident classification system (Resource Utilization Groups III) based on data from resident assessments (MDS 2.0, mentioned in Chapter 6) and relative weights developed from staff time data. This information is extremely detailed and is presently undergoing changes that are expected to become effective in 2001. The reader is recommended to visit the AOTA and HCFA websites for additional and current information related to PPS in SNFs and other areas of practice.

Medicaid

Medicaid or Medical Assistance is a state government funded program for low-income families and individuals. Programs are managed individually by each state and states are increasingly using HMOs to implement the Medicaid programs. States follow individual sets of guidelines but all require only participation by providers with credentials equal to those required for the state's licensure, certification, and/or national regulatory board (this is true for all fiscal agencies). See Appendix A-3.2 for a list of state licensing and regulatory agencies.

Once a provider number is given, the provider should receive a participation manual outlining requirements for participation, documentation, claims submission information, specific coding, prior authorization, and durable medical equipment (DME) coverage. For further detail about state-to-state regulations refer to the Health Care Financing Administration (HCFA) at www.hcfa.gov/medicaid/.

Generally, policies may allow a specified number of treatment sessions per calendar year before preauthorization (PA) is required, but some programs suggest submitting a PA before evaluation and treatment is begun to assure approval. This is because often occupational therapy services from all providers are included in the total per year. There is also a limit on the number of times an evaluation will be approved in the same calendar year, for the same diagnosis, and on the number of same or similar DME disbursed annually.

Children's Services

In addition to Medicaid, many states have alternative funding and rules for children's services. HCFA posts information related to the State Children's

Health Insurance Program (SCHIP), or Title XXI, which was passed as part of the BBA of 1997. States that have submitted state plans to access the funds authorized under Title XXI are listed at www.hcfa.gov/init/statepln.htm.

State plans are available from officials listed on the website.

The insurance commission offices in each state are also excellent resources for guidance about children's and other health insurance plans in the state. A listing of the 2000 insurance commissioners' offices can be found in Appendix A-7.2.

Supplemental Insurance

Medicare coverage for recipients covers 80 percent of "allowable" or approved expenses. This means if $40.00 was charged for the procedure and Medicare allows $28.00 for that service, they will pay 80 percent of $28.00, or $22.40.

If the provider accepts Medicare "assignment," this means they will receive that amount and cannot bill the uncovered portion to the consumer. If the provider does not accept assignment, they will have a lower "allowable" payment, but they can shift the non-covered charges to the consumer.

To receive payment for the remaining 20 percent, the recipient has the option to purchase supplementary insurance, such as Medigap, or one of the numerous other options. If the income level of the insured meets certain criteria, the individual may qualify for Medicaid as a secondary carrier.

The supplemental policy, with the exception of Medicaid for some procedures, only pays for the remainder of what Medicare has already *allowed*. In other words, most policies will not cover services provided if Medicare denies the claim as a non-covered service. In the previous example, the secondary policy would pay 20 percent of the $28.00, or $5.60. It is very rare to find a secondary policy that will cover everything that Medicare does not pay, but this is usually very confusing to the recipient. It should be explained carefully, as many consumers believe their supplemental policy will pay anything that Medicare does not. If there is a question, it is always better to call the carrier to confirm the payment policy.

Worker's Compensation

Work related injuries comprise another sector of health care for which OTs provide service and are reimbursed. Worker's compensation programs are governed by individual states and may employ case managers (sometimes OTs) and rehabilitation nurses to be involved in coordinating the care for injured workers.

Frequently, it is the case manager who approves the services and claims for the injured employee. Therefore, the case manager becomes a consumer to the OT, in addition to the worker. Good communication about the treatment plan, anticipated changes, treatment progress, and outcomes will facilitate payment for services provided. The case manager is also a source of new referrals and should be sought out by the therapist if there is one placed on the case. This is determined by contacting the worker's compensation carrier if the case manager does not make contact first.

It is recommended that all care and equipment be approved prior to implementation and billing. Coordinating efforts with the employer for work adaptations, restrictions, and return to work, if necessary, promotes overall reduction in health care costs, and is usually supported by the worker's compensation carrier.

Billing for OT Services

Submitting claims to insurance carriers for OT services is done using claim forms designed by the Health Care Financing Administration (HCFA). Two forms are widely accepted (and required for some claims submission), and are chosen depending upon the type of setting in which services are provided. The HCFA-1500 is used for private OT clinics and outpatient settings, the HCFA-1450 (UB-92) is used for inpatient hospital stays. (See Figures 7.1 and 7.2) These documents are for viewing only and not for reproduction or actual use. The reader is directed to the web address www.hcfa.gov/forms/default.asp, which gives instructions for completing forms, downloading, printing, or receiving electronic HCFA forms free of charge. Any question whether these forms are current should be resolved by contacting HCFA or the appropriate HCFA contractor.

Please note that some states do not accept black and white copies of these forms, and the figures included for the purposes of this text are not formatted correctly. The reader is recommended to obtain actual copies for use at the website referenced above, or order electronic copy.

The National Uniform Billing Committee was responsible for the national uniform billing system (UB-92) and its manual, and paper forms are available from the Standard Register, Forms Division, at 1-800-755-6405.

The American Medical Association (AMA) and other sources publish and maintain a listing and description of services and procedures performed by physicians and non-physician practitioners, known as the current procedural terminology (CPT) codebook: CPT-4. CPT codes are required by most third-party payers including Medicare and Medical Assistance when billing for OT services. It is incumbent upon the practitioner to remain informed of current policy regulations, variations in individual payer policy, and differences in state regulations. Although the CPT codebook is updated, revised, and published annually, some carriers recognize other more dated versions. The AMA and St. Anthony's Press are among the publishers for this book. It is not published on the Internet, but ordering information can be obtained at www.aota.org in the reimbursement section.

The present use of CPT codes specific to OT services includes:

- the 95000 section for neurology and neuromuscular procedures
- the 96000 section for central nervous systems assessments and tests
- the 97000 section for physical medicine and rehabilitation procedures

Codes are typically based on fifteen-minute units and should be billed accordingly unless otherwise noted in the current CPT codebook; e.g., work hardening is billed in initial two-hour segments and every hour subsequently. Some codes are considered "non timed" per service codes and are reimbursed per procedure without regard to time, e.g., evaluation.

When determining which code describes the treatment performed, the therapist must be able to justify its use and have documentation to support the procedure billed. Procedure modifiers are added to the five-digit CPT code when the service provided is substantially different from the code description. If a modifier is used, a report should be attached to the bill. Some CPT codes frequently used by OTs cannot be billed simultaneously without a modifier.

Use published CPT codebooks and/or the AOTA reimbursement department web page for additional coding procedures..

In addition to the CPT procedural code, a diagnosis code called International Classification of Diseases, 9th Revision, Clinical Modification (ICD-9 CM) is used to indicate consumer diagnosis, suggesting a reason for the service provided. A treatment diagnosis, which is interpreted to mean "the

PLEASE
DO NOT
STAPLE
IN THIS
AREA

(SAMPLE ONLY - NOT APPROVED FOR USE)

CARRIER

☐☐ PICA   **HEALTH INSURANCE CLAIM FORM**   PICA ☐☐

| 1. MEDICARE   MEDICAID   CHAMPUS   CHAMPVA   GROUP HEALTH PLAN   FECA BLK LUNG   OTHER | 1a. INSURED'S I.D. NUMBER   (FOR PROGRAM IN ITEM 1) |
| ☐ (Medicare #) ☐ (Medicaid #) ☐ (Sponsor's SSN) ☐ (VA File #) ☐ (SSN or ID) ☐ (SSN) ☐ (ID) | |

| 2. PATIENT'S NAME (Last Name, First Name, Middle Initial) | 3. PATIENT'S BIRTH DATE   SEX | 4. INSURED'S NAME (Last Name, First Name, Middle Initial) |
| | MM ¦ DD ¦ YY   M☐ F☐ | |

| 5. PATIENT'S ADDRESS (No. Street) | 6. PATIENT RELATIONSHIP TO INSURED | 7. INSURED'S ADDRESS (No. Street) |
| | Self ☐ Spouse ☐ Child ☐ Other ☐ | |

| CITY   STATE | 8. PATIENT STATUS | CITY   STATE |
| | Single ☐ Married ☐ Other ☐ | |

| ZIP CODE   TELEPHONE (Include Area Code) (   ) | Employed ☐ Full-Time Student ☐ Part-Time Student ☐ | ZIP CODE   TELEPHONE (INCLUDE AREA CODE) (   ) |

| 9. OTHER INSURED'S NAME (Last Name, First Name, Middle Initial) | 10. IS PATIENT'S CONDITION RELATED TO: | 11. INSURED'S POLICY GROUP OR FECA NUMBER |

| a. OTHER INSURED'S POLICY OR GROUP NUMBER | a. EMPLOYMENT? (CURRENT OR PREVIOUS) ☐ YES ☐ NO | a. INSURED'S DATE OF BIRTH   SEX MM ¦ DD ¦ YY   M☐ F☐ |

| b. OTHER INSURED'S DATE OF BIRTH   SEX MM ¦ DD ¦ YY   M☐ F☐ | b. AUTO ACCIDENT?   PLACE (State) ☐ YES ☐ NO | b. EMPLOYER'S NAME OR SCHOOL NAME |

| c. EMPLOYER'S NAME OR SCHOOL NAME | c. OTHER ACCIDENT? ☐ YES ☐ NO | c. INSURANCE PLAN NAME OR PROGRAM NAME |

| d. INSURANCE PLAN NAME OR PROGRAM NAME | 10d. RESERVED FOR LOCAL USE | d. IS THERE ANOTHER HEALTH BENEFIT PLAN? ☐ YES ☐ NO If yes, return to and complete item 9 a – d. |

READ BACK OF FORM BEFORE COMPLETING & SIGNING THIS FORM.

| 12. PATIENT'S OR AUTHORIZED PERSON'S SIGNATURE I authorize the release of any medical or other information necessary to process this claim. I also request payment of government benefits either to myself or to the party who accepts assignment below.   SIGNED _____   DATE _____ | 13. INSURED'S OR AUTHORIZED PERSON'S SIGNATURE I authorize payment of medical benefits to the undersigned physician or supplier for services described below.   SIGNED _____ |

PATIENT AND INSURED INFORMATION

| 14. DATE OF CURRENT: ILLNESS (First symptom) OR MM ¦ DD ¦ YY ◄ INJURY (Accident) OR PREGNANCY (LMP) | 15. IF PATIENT HAS HAD SAME OR SIMILAR ILLNESS, GIVE FIRST DATE   MM ¦ DD ¦ YY | 16. DATES PATIENT UNABLE TO WORK IN CURRENT OCCUPATION MM ¦ DD ¦ YY   MM ¦ DD ¦ YY FROM   TO |

| 17. NAME OF REFERRING PHYSICIAN OR OTHER SOURCE | 17a. I.D. NUMBER OF REFERRING PHYSICIAN | 18. HOSPITALIZATION DATES RELATED TO CURRENT SERVICES MM ¦ DD ¦ YY   MM ¦ DD ¦ YY FROM   TO |

| 19. RESERVED FOR LOCAL USE | | 20. OUTSIDE LAB? $ CHARGES ☐ YES ☐ NO |

21. DIAGNOSIS OR NATURE OF ILLNESS OR INJURY. (RELATE ITEMS 1, 2, 3, OR 4 TO ITEM 24E BY LINE)	22. MEDICAID RESUBMISSION CODE ORIGINAL REF. NO.
1. L___ . ___ 3. L___ . ___	
2. L___ . ___ 4. L___ . ___	23. PRIOR AUTHORIZATION NUMBER

24. A. DATE(S) OF SERVICE		B. Place of Service	C. Type of Service	D. PROCEDURES, SERVICES, OR SUPPLIES (Explain Unusual Circumstances) CPT/HCPCS MODIFIER	E. DIAGNOSIS CODE	F. $ CHARGES	G. DAYS OR UNITS	H. EPSDT Family Plan	I. EMG	J. COB	K. RESERVED FOR LOCAL USE
From MM DD YY	To MM DD YY										
1											
2											
3											
4											
5											
6											

| 25. FEDERAL TAX I.D. NUMBER   SSN ☐ EIN ☐ | 26. PATIENT'S ACCOUNT NO. | 27. ACCEPT ASSIGNMENT? (For govt. claims, see back) ☐ YES ☐ NO | 28. TOTAL CHARGE $ | 29. AMOUNT PAID $ | 30. BALANCE DUE $ |

| 31. SIGNATURE OF PHYSICIAN OR SUPPLIER INCLUDING DEGREES OR CREDENTIALS (I certify that the statements on the reverse apply to this bill and are made a part thereof.)   SIGNED _____   DATE _____ | 32. NAME AND ADDRESS OF FACILITY WHERE SERVICES WERE RENDERED (If other than home or office) | 33. PHYSICIAN'S SUPPLIER'S BILLING NAME, ADDRESS, ZIP CODE & PHONE #   PIN#   GRP# |

PHYSICIAN OR SUPPLIER INFORMATION

(SAMPLE ONLY - NOT APPROVED FOR USE)   *PLEASE PRINT OR TYPE*   SAMPLE FORM 1500
                                                                                SAMPLE FORM 1500 SAMPLE FORM 1500

Figure 7.1. HCFA-1500 Form

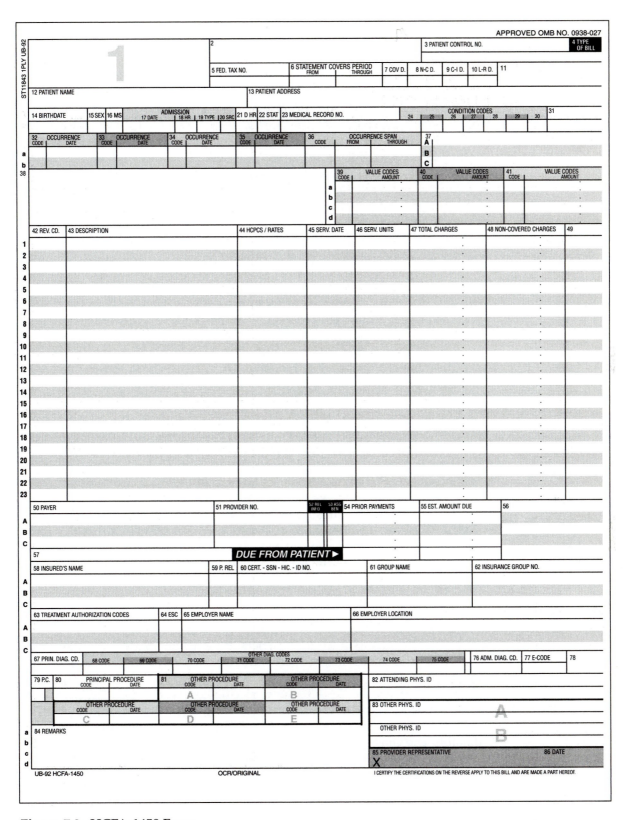

Figure 7.2. HCFA-1450 Form

diagnosis for which treatment is being requested," is also listed on the HCFA form. In other words, a consumer is not seeking OT services because they had a stroke, but because they now may have right upper extremity hemiparesis, decreased functional ability, and/or shoulder pain, for example. Chronic conditions are listed on the HCFA form only if relevant to services offered.

St. Anthony's Press as well as the American Medical Association and other publishers publish ICD-9 code books. These code books are also updated annually. These codes can also be found at www.mcis.duke.edu/standards/termcode/icd9/1tabular.html. The ICD-9 will be replaced in the near future with the 10th edition of this coding system, the ICD-10.

For Medicare Part B recipients, only the diagnosis codes (ICD-9 codes) listed for each procedure in the PHYSMED-009 are reimbursed, while other ICD-9 codes that are not listed are considered to be non-covered according to the policy.

The AOTA summarizes the HCPCS, pronounced hics pics (HCFA Common Procedure Coding System), in the *Elements of Clinical Documentation*, Thomson, L.K. & Foto, M. (1995) publication available to AOTA members. Information about HCPCS can also be obtained at www.hcfa.gov/medicare/hcpcs.htm. The HCPCS coding system consists of three levels. They include the Level 1 CPT code, and the Level 2 national "alpha numeric" codes developed by HCFA for services and supplies for which no CPT code exists. These codes are used to bill for durable medical equipment (DME), orthotics, prosthetics, and supplies, and can be found in a separate HCPCS code book. Level 3 codes are the local codes developed by HCFA carriers to describe new procedures and supplies for which no Level 1 or 2 codes exist (AOTA, 1998).

A facility may bill using the 1450 form (UB-92) for Medicare Part A and DME supplies (Appendix A-7.3). Private providers must apply for a DME provider number to bill Medicare for these supplies, including splints and orthotics.

Another coding system used for claims submission is known as the Diagnostic and Statistical Manual of Mental Disorders, fourth edition (DSM-IV). It is a classification system used for sixteen major diagnostic classes of mental disorders (i.e., substance-related disorders, anxiety disorders, mood disorders, eating disorders) and is commonly used by mental health professionals. The DSM-IV is coordinated closely with Chapter IV, "mental and behavioral disorders," of the ICD-9 system.

Private Payers

With over 200 private insurance carriers in the United States, reimbursement for OT services is dependent upon each payer's individual policies and regulations. These vary between carriers and even within the same company of multi-state programs. To determine specific coverage for OT services, each payer needs to be addressed directly regarding individual insurance plans.

Consumer insurance cards will identify telephone numbers for benefit coordinators, and can be used for specific coverage questions. This department can also provide general coverage information for each insurance carrier. Getting preauthorization for services prior to commencing services is a good practice (see later this chapter).

Billing Tips and Suggestions

A combination of medical and treatment diagnoses are used when submitting a claim for occupational therapy services and should be as specific as possible. Documentation for each claim should be available for review by the payer if requested. Each procedure billed is described in daily documentation as provided as related to the condition or diagnosis using wording included in the CPT procedure to ensure payment. The payer will target functional deficits and improvements in any medical review, therefore, inclusion in documentation is necessary.

AOTA offers significant in-depth information about reimbursement at their website www.aota.org. Members are provided with reimbursement decision guides and algorithms for each area of practice, with the use of a password obtained at the website. Links to many pertinent agencies also exist here. Readers are strongly encouraged to look to these documents for detailed information about reimbursement procedures in specific practice settings.

Medicare resources include:

- Home Health Prospective Payment System (PPS) Final Rule (HCFA1059-F), 6-28-2000.
- PPS for Hospital Outpatient Services, 3-31-00.
- Medicare Provider Reimbursement Manual.
  - HCFA Pub 15-1
  - Order #PB 97-954800
  - Describes reimbursement to hospitals and SNFs under the PPS. Outlines payment system for providers qualifying for reimbursement using a reasonable cost basis.
- Medicare Intermediary Manual, Audits, Reimbursement, Program Administration, Pt. 2.
  - Provides intermediaries with instructions for claiming reimbursement and time frames for processing claims
- Medicare Intermediary Manual, Claims Process, Pt. 3.
  - Pub 13-3
  - #99-95460
  - Contains instruction and procedures for processing claims, including coverage limitations and coverage requirements.
    - The beneficiary appeals process included.

Again, go to www.hcfa.gov/regs/regsnotices.htm.

Other Reimbursement Alternatives

For many years, in many scopes of practice, payment for the services provided by occupational therapists were included in the patient or resident room rate or program cost. This method of payment may continue to be a viable alternative into the future if the importance of OT as members of the "team" can be justified.

If OT is to be billed as an "overhead charge," it will be because the service is felt to be *needed* for the positive outcome of the overall program. OTs must be able to justify their necessity, clarify their roles, and be confident in their identity as members of the health care, workforce, or educational team.

Effectiveness can be established through outcomes data and documented case studies. For more detailed information about collecting data and implementing outcome studies, see Chapter 8 entitled Outcomes Research.

Community agencies, federal waiver programs, and private support groups offer many alternatives for payment of OT services when traditional third party payment is unavailable. County human and social service departments, federal waiver programs, Native American tribal funds, groups such as the

Multiple Sclerosis Association, United Cerebral Palsy, the Muscular Dystrophy Association, to name a few, are sometimes able to provide payment for equipment and/or treatment provided by an occupational therapist or occupational therapy assistant.

Denials and Appeals

There are times when a payer denies a claim for services billed. The fiscal agency needs to provide a reason for denial on the explanation of benefits (EOB) report received, which describes claims and dates submitted, payments made, and payments allowed.

Each payer has a specific policy to appeal a denial. Additional documentation must be submitted describing the medical necessity of treatment and justification of the need for procedures provided. The Medicare appeals process can be found in the Intermediary Manual Part 3 Chapter VIII—Payment Procedures, beginning at section 3799 and found at www.hcfa.gov/pub-forms/13%5Fint/a3799.htm.

It is important to note that providers have a legal obligation to advocate for the health care needs of their consumers and may be potentially liable if they do not. Therefore fiscal intermediaries and carriers need to be targeted with documentation in support of payment and coverage of medically necessary services as appropriate to the consumer.

Preauthorization

Although it is ultimately the responsibility of the consumer to understand the benefits of their insurance policy, therapists and therapy managers are recommended to determine coverage prior to treatment implementation. This is accomplished by calling the fiscal intermediary of government programs, the case manager, or insurance carrier with the consumer's Social Security number, birth date, and group or plan number.

The reader is referred to state policies for Medicaid prior authorization, as stated earlier in the chapter.

Summary

Because continued evolution of payment strategies are imminent, the occupational therapist must be informed of current legislation affecting health care; specifically, reimbursement of rehabilitation services. It is also incumbent upon the therapist to be informed of correct coding and billing procedures to maximize reimbursement. This places the OT in a new role, one of:

- Understanding the requirements of the payer for documentation and coverage services
- Being proactive in providing efficient services with positive outcomes
- Communicating with the payer about treatment plans and expectations for progress
- Becoming a member of participating health care plans by contacting each payer individually

With this type of organization and practice, occupational therapy services should continue to be reimbursable and OT will remain a viable member of the health care team.

CHAPTER 8

Outcomes Research

Outcome measurement is a method used to evaluate the effectiveness of health care procedures, including occupational therapy. To be successful in marketing the skills of occupational therapists as team members, program participants, and/or consultants, OT must substantiate the value of their services. By researching the benefit of OT for the consumer, occupational therapists are more likely to be acknowledged as necessary contributors to the care of the consumer. "The challenges facing occupational therapists include proving our value in an economic trend of downsizing, competing within the medical profession, developing and affiliating with new payer sources, and reengineering our careers to meet the needs of the new, nontraditional health care marketplace" (Ellenberg, 1996).

Measuring outcomes in health care is not a new concept, but has come to the forefront of many practice models as accountability and cost containment became a national trend. The use of outcome measurement in nontraditional settings, however, has not become common practice and, therefore, it is incumbent upon occupational therapists to be leaders in this area. By providing results of treatment protocol effectiveness and measures of the contribution of OT on cost containment, the opportunities for OTs are likely to expand as a greater value is placed on the skills that an occupational therapist possesses.

At the conclusion of this chapter, the reader will be able to:

1. Discuss basic concepts related to the need for measuring outcomes in occupational therapy.

2. Understand the steps for establishing an outcomes measurement system.

3. Know the types of indicators appropriate for OT programs.

4. Understand tools for measuring and monitoring outcomes.

Outcome Measurement

Outcomes are defined in many different ways as they relate to measurement of success in health care delivery. Jenkinson (1994) describes outcomes in terms of mortality, morbidity, physiological measures, and the patient's subjective assessment of health. In other words, they are the end result of medical interventions according to Jenkinson. An outcome is more simply defined by the New South Wales Health Department (1992), p. 135, as "a change in the health of an individual, group of people or population, which is attributable to an intervention, or series of interventions."

Outcome measurement uses a strategic method of collecting data about the effectiveness of treatment techniques, cost effectiveness of programs, and assessment of health care quality of life. Using outcome measurement in OT has other benefits. Clinical decision making, strategies, and treatment techniques may be adjusted based on results. The effectiveness of a treatment technique, protocol, or time frame can be established. Marketing, program justification, reimbursement, provider status, and policy setting can all be addressed as a result of outcome studies. Treatment plans can be adjusted, and therapy continued or discontinued. Any positive results obtained should be communicated to consumers, including payers, referral sources, administrators, and the public to substantiate the benefit of occupational therapy services.

Pryzybylski, B. R., et al. (1996) produced an outcome study that substantiates the benefits of OT. They concluded that increasing the amounts of OT and physical therapy (PT) can have positive effects on the functional status of long-term care nursing home residents and showed a cost savings of $283 per bed annually. The Functional Independence Measure (FIM), Functional Assessment Measures (FAM), and Clinical Outcomes Variable Scale (COVS) were used as tools to gather data.

Indicators

Outcome measurement indicators can be developed for most any area of the therapy process. "Indicators" are the factors to be studied and can be derived with input from the consumer, caregiver, and/or therapist.

Indicators to consider when implementing an outcomes research program for an OT department are:

- Functional independence
- Musculoskeletal factors; i.e., range of motion, strength, edema
- Work-employment status, i.e., return to work, work placement, amount of on-the-job assistance required
- Patient satisfaction
- Prevention or need for surgical intervention
- Pain
- Sensation
- Manual dexterity
- Supported living needs
- Emotional-behavioral status
- Medication intake
- Cost of services
- Duration, Length, and Frequency of Treatment

Because many of these indicators are already used routinely in the occupational therapist's evaluation/reevaluation, implementing an outcomes research program may be as simple as establishing a data collection system. For example, a department interested in determining the impact of a pain management program may choose to compile results of all pain scales initially and upon discharge. The data is then analyzed for cumulative results.

Developing an Outcomes Measurement System

Munro (as cited in Mayhan, 1994) describes some of the concepts below for developing an outcome measurement system:

1. Determine what information the consumer, payer, administrator, etc. are seeking.

2. Start with simple strategies that will allow the program manager to obtain results, which can be analyzed and implemented in short periods of time. (More detailed studies can follow at a later date as needed.)

3. Use measurement tools that have already been established, if possible.

4. Consider use of professional researchers as consultants for new study development. There are companies that set up programs for data collection of specified indicators.

5. Access regional or national databases to reinforce the justification of occupational therapy services to payers and administrators.

6. Capitalize on positive outcomes that address negative findings. Always adjust the system to improve quality.

7. Implement methods of emphasizing the unique features of the therapy program.

8. Involve all staff in carrying out the chosen measurement system. This will create ownership and encourage active problem solving.

Data Collection Tools

Many instruments are available for data collection. The level of sophistication of the desired results will determine the tool chosen to assess the outcome. For research projects, it is important to find out if the instrument has been previously used in a similar setting and what the validity of the instrument is for that situation. This information can be found in databases such as MEDLINE or the Outcomes Activities Database at the library.

Many systems offer detailed statistical programs for data retrieval and interpretation. Others offer computer software capability for ease in statistical calculations. A few of the many options available to the occupational therapy manager are described below.

1. Canadian Occupational Performance Measure (COPM) is a standardized instrument developed by occupational therapists to be used as an outcome measure. It has undergone significant research in a variety of practice areas. This tool detects a consumer's self-perceived change in their occupational performance over time. The following web page provides further information by visiting www.caot.ca/copm/.

2. The Uniform Data System for Medical Rehabilitation (UDSMR) uses reporting software to document restorative/rehabilitative efficiency and effectiveness. Included are performance measures for:

   • Hospital medical rehabilitation programs for adults

   • Hospital medical rehabilitation programs for pediatrics

   • Long-term care facilities for adult restorative patients

   • Long-term care facilities for pediatric restorative patients

   • Behavioral health care organizations for pediatrics (in development)

   • Ambulatory care for pediatrics (in development)

3. OT Fact (Occupational Therapy Functional Assessment Compilation Tool) is a collection and reporting system for functional performance tasks. As stated in Chapter 6, Documentation, it is able to compile data sequentially over time of OT intervention. Software programs are available through: www.execpc.com/~dgtldesn/otfact.htm.

4. The Functional Independence Measure (FIM)™ (Guide for the Uniform Data Set for Medical Rehabilitation, 1996) is a widely accepted assessment of functional skills and provides uniform measurement of disability and rehabilitation outcomes. It was developed with sponsorship from the American Congress of Rehabilitation Medicine and the American Academy of Physical Medicine and Rehabilitation, according to Granger et al., 1986. In 1990 Granger determined that the precision of the FIM was high. More information about the FIM can be obtained from www.tbims.org/combi/FIM/.

5. Medicare OASIS: the Outcome and Assessment Information Set for Home Health Care is an example of an extensive outcome measurement tool in home health care. It targets areas such as living arrangements, supportive assistance, sensory status, integumentary status, respiratory status, elimination status, neuro-emotional-behavioral status, activities of daily living and instrumental activities of daily living, medications, equipment management, and emergent care for determination of program effectiveness. Further information can be obtained at www.hcfa.gov/medical/oasis/oasishmp.htm.

6. The Level of Rehabilitation Scale (Lors-III Reference Manual, 1994) is a national database for program evaluation and outcome comparison in rehabilitation. Information about ADL and cognitive performance can be assessed using the Lors-III. Velozo, Pan, Magalhaes, and Leiter, 1995 analyzed its effectiveness.

7. Patient Evaluation and Conference System (PECS™) is a rehabilitation outcomes reporting system to gather initial through discharge status. It was initially introduced at the University of Wisconsin-Madison in 1979 and has been continually developed with the support of the Marion Joy Rehabilitation Network, Wheaton, Illinois. More information can be found at www.rfi.org.

8. The SF-36 is a general measure of Health Related Quality of Life (HRQL) (Ware & Sherbourne, 1992). It is copyrighted and distributed by MOS Trust, 20 Park Plaza, Suite 1014 Boston, MA 12116-4313. Telephone: 617-426-4046/ Fax: 617-426-4131/ email: motrust@worldnet.att.net. Reliability and validity was addressed by Ware, J.E. 2000. More information can be found at www.sf-36.com.

9. The Functional Status Questionnaire (FSQ)(Jette, et al. 1986) is an assessment tool used to obtain information about the physical, psychological, social, and role function in ambulatory individuals. A study about the reliability and validity of this instrument when used in primary care has been completed by Jette et al., 1986. More information can be obtained at www.qlmed.org/fsq/index.html.

10. The Nottingham Health Profile (NHP)(McEwen, 1998) is another general health status questionnaire and can be obtained from Galen Research, Southern Hey, Barlow Moor Road, West Didsbury, Manchester, M20 8PW, UK. Telephone: 44-161-448-1600, fax: 44-161-446-2544.

11. The upper extremity network (UE NET) is a national outcomes database created by the American Society of Hand Therapists (ASHT) and the American Society of Surgery of the Hand. This tool measures outcomes specific to hand and upper extremity rehabilitation.

12. For assessment of the spine, lower extremity, and upper extremity in regards to effectiveness of treatment, the Dexter System and Treatment Outcome Program offers a software tracking system. Calculations for range of motion, skeletal examinations, whole body impairments, and an HRQL Assessment (SF-36) are among its capabilities.

13. The ORCA is a software application specific to the upper extremity and hand. It is compatible with the Newton Personal Digital Assistant, which is a hand-held computer used in clinical situations. ORCA is designed to allow clinics participating in the upper extremity net to input data with greater ease. It was also created with a focus on meeting the needs of managed care systems. ORCA is manufactured by Greenleaf Medical Systems, 2248 Park Boulevard, Palo Alto, California 94306.

14. The Cognitive Performance Scale (CPS) was developed to describe cognitive status using items from the Minimum Data Set (MDS) instrument. It combines information on memory impairment, level of consciousness, and executive function.

15. WeeFIM system measures functional performance in self-care, mobility, and cognitive areas for individuals ages 6 months to 18 to 21 years. It documents functional outcomes across inpatient, outpatient, and community settings. 716-829-2076, info@weefim.org.

The Clearing House Health Outcomes, www.leeds.ac.uk/nuffield/infoservices/UKCH/define.html, presents a significant amount of outcomes measurement information. A biannual publication, *Outcomes Briefing*, from the UK Clearing House provides valuable information to the researcher interested in outcomes. The following topics are addressed individually in files that can be obtained at www.leeds.ac.uk/nuffield/infoservices/UKCH/publi.html:

1. An introduction to measuring health outcomes

2. Multidimensional profiles

3. Searching the outcomes literature

4. Review of the SF-36

5. Exploring outcomes within routine practice

6. Broadening the base for outcomes measurement: criteria for selecting measures

7. Outcomes within clinical audit

8. Outcomes, patients, and caregivers

In addition, the UK Clearing House has an outcomes measurement review series on topics relevant to the OT. They include guidelines for studying total hip replacements, alcohol misuse, and stroke care, to name a few. This information is also available at the website referenced above.

Internet and Other References for Outcome Measurement

- Cochran Collaboration http://hiru.mcmaster.ca/cochrane/default.htm
- European Clearing Houses on Health Outcomes (ECHHO)
  www.leeds.ac.uk/nuffield/infoservices/ecchho/home.html
- Medical Outcomes Trust www.outcomes-trust.org
- University of Sheffield—Scharr School of Health and Related Research
  www.shef.ac.uk/uni/academic/R-Z/scharr/research.htm

- Supporting Clinical Outcomes in Primary Care for the Elderly (SCOPE) www.otworks.com

Summary

The use of outcomes measurement and management will continue to be an important aspect in occupational therapy programming. It is included in the measurement standards required of accreditations agencies. Its benefits are multifaceted: evaluation of patient satisfaction, treatment effectiveness, appropriate therapy interventions, and quality of care are the most obvious. Improvements in clinical decision making, marketing, contract negotiations, and accountability are often secondary benefits.

Occupational therapy managers should be alert to the need to substantiate the value of occupational therapy with a strategic outcome measurement system. Through data collection and communication of findings, the position of occupational therapists can be strengthened within the health care delivery system, in addition to nontraditional practice settings.

Case Study 1

An occupational therapy department in an inpatient mental health facility would like to determine the effectiveness of purposeful activity with its consumers.

Discussion Questions

1. What indicator could be studied?
2. Set up a measurement collection technique for the therapist(s) to use with their consumers.
3. Are there any outcome studies established for this type of program? If so, which one(s) would be appropriate for this setting?
4. How could an outcomes research program benefit the consumers, therapist, and OT department?
5. What measurement tool would be appropriate for this study?

CHAPTER 9

Technology in Occupational Therapy

Abundant technological advances have been made in health care and education since the computer era began. Available to the occupational therapist today are computer programs and tools for evaluation, treatment, adaptations, billing, communication, transcription, research, and education. Ability to access information via the World Wide Web has significantly increased ease and abundance of resources. Internet services offer a mode of communication for information transmittal and retrieval, in addition to marketing and advertisement.

Assistive technology was once an adjunct to occupational therapy treatment techniques, but has developed into an immense field in and of itself. Specialty certification is available in this area. Public education has adopted assistive technology guidelines in special needs programming. The need for the occupational therapist to be aware of these resources is obvious.

Technology in the Office

Office management is made easier due to the advances of technology for communication, billing, and documentation. To stay abreast of changes, the occupational therapy manager is encouraged to be informed of the many opportunities available which can save time and money when implementing the office management systems.

Electronic Billing

Advances in claims submission progressed from handwritten, to computer generated, to paperless claims in a relatively short period of time. Electronic billing is the preferred method by many reimbursement sources, e.g., insurance companies, including Medicare and Medicaid. Eventually nearly all bills for medical services will be submitted electronically.

The initial step in filing claims via the Internet is to choose a type of medical billing software that has the appropriate compatibilities. There are many companies selling software for medical billing. Software prices vary from approximately $1,000 to $10,000, depending on amenities included. Standard programs include, but are not limited to, scheduling, invoicing, and month-end reports. Outcome tracking, medical record keeping, home care input, free clearinghouse charges, and free training are available depending upon the program. See Figure 9.1 for a vendor list including some medical billing software companies.

The second step is to choose a clearinghouse. Although any clearinghouse can be used, the billing software company may acknowledge the program warranty only if the one they suggest is enrolled. The clearinghouse charges a fee for each claim submitted, although this fee may vary. The insurance companies to be billed must be listed with the clearinghouse in order to submit the claims electronically. The clearinghouse will forward this list to the provider prior to enrollment, to determine if the insurance companies typically billed by the provider are accessible by the clearinghouse. If not, a more compatible clearinghouse must be chosen.

The next step is to receive permission to file claims electronically from Medicare, Medicaid, and any other insurance carriers. The billing software company can provide the paperwork to request permission from identified carriers. In some cases the request is then submitted to the national clearinghouse, which, in turn, submits the request to the payer. This process can take a minimum of four to six weeks. When permission has been received from a carrier, the process is then completed and claims can be filed electronically.

When a claim is submitted in this manner, it is initially transmitted to the clearinghouse for review. If omissions or errors exist, a rejection is received by the provider. "Clean claims" (claims without errors) are forwarded to the carrier within 24 hours of receipt by the clearinghouse.

Although the initial process of enrollment appears cumbersome, when the process is implemented, a huge savings can be realized in office staff and wages over time. Filing electronic claims is extremely energy efficient and payment is expedited as a result.

As expected, software programs are available for diagnostic and procedure coding as well. Large facilities with billing departments operate with this type of system and often have a person(s) to fill this role. Using a search key for difficult diagnoses shaves minutes and hours off time spent paging through a book.

Technology in Documentation

In most cases, voice activated dictation programs are not sophisticated enough to handle the demands of occupational therapy reports. The downfalls exist in the limited capability of the system to integrate the information accurately as it is dictated. Eventually, these programs will be perfected and used widely among occupational therapists for dictation purposes. Presently, most dictation is done through manual dictation systems implementing the use of a transcriptionist to type reports.

New technology has allowed for the use of dictation systems which are designed to transmit voice recordings electronically to another computer for transcription purposes. This offers the therapist the opportunity to dictate reports from other locations.

Software for Financial Management

Accounting software programs are commonplace for business, as well as home computers. Expenses and revenues can be tracked and reports generated such as cash flow status, balance sheets, and profit and loss statements. Checks can be printed and payroll completed with the use of such programs. Detailed payroll reports can be generated and vendor lists complied.

Assistive Technology and Equipment

(This is not intended to be a practitioner's list but to begin the "linking" process.)

1. AbleNet, Inc.
   www.ablenetinc.com

2. Adaptive and Assistive Technology
   www.RehabTool.com

3. Adaptive Engineering Lab, Inc.
   www.aelseating.com

4. Aurora Systems, Inc.
   www.djtech.com/aurora/

5. Better Life Online Catalogue
   www.traveller.com/dymedias

6. Miscellaneous web addresses
   (AOTA web site-Assistive Tech SIS)

   a. www.accessunlimited.com

   b. http://www.members.tripod.com/
      gobrowns/devices.htm

   c. www.bv.net/~john/bethsotl.html

   d. www.childrenwithdisabilities.ncjrs.org/

   e. http://www.clinweb2.kumc.edu/

   f. www.naotd.org/linklink.htm

   g. www.atnet.org

Strengthening, Function, Prosthetics, and Work Performance

1. Baltimore Theraputic Equipment (BTE)
   www.bteco.com/

2. Biometrics, Ltd.
   www.biometricsltd.com

3. 3D Static Strength Prediction Program
   (University of Michigan)
   www.engin.umich.edu/dept/ioe/3DSSPP/

4. Key Assessment

5. Biodex Medical Systems
   www.biodex.com

Accounting Software Programs

1. Absolute Business Software
   www.channel1.com.users/abs/

2. Accounting Information Systems
   www.aissf.com/

3. Accounting Store
   www.accountingstore.com/

4. Asset Business Software
   www.grailworks.com/abs/intro.htp

5. Brickell Research
   www.brickellresearch.com/

6. Quickbooks
   www.intuit.com/quickbooks/

7. 247 Software: Small Business and Accounting Software
   www.247software.net/smallbusiness.htm

8. 2000 Accounting
   www.2000accounting.com/

Medical Billing Software

1. Clarisys 35
   www.clarisys.ca/free.html

2. Cougar Mountain Software
   www.cougarmtn.com/

3. Gateway Technologies
   www.gatewaytech.com/meddent.htm

4. KIP Medical Billing Software
   www.kipdeluxe.com/

5. MacHealth Medical Manager
   www.healthcc.com/

6. Medisoft: Affordable Billing Software
   www.medicalbillingprogram.com/

7. Mesonic Software Services
   www.Mesonic.com/

8. National Data Corp
   www.ndcorp.com/

Figure 9.1 Technology Vendor List *Please Note: The intended use of this list of vendors is for reference only. The products included are in no way endorsed by this publisher or author.*

In many cases, use of an accounting software program can save the occupational therapy manager time and money while increasing organizational skills and generating valuable reports. Often the accountant used for the practice will have compatible software, and changes to the business accounts can be done easily through disc exchange. This is a very convenient method of monthly account balancing. See Figure 9.1 for a list of vendors including accounting software programs.

On-line Communication and Continuing Education

With the presence of electronic mail, more commonly known as e-mail, an additional mode of communication has been introduced to the world. Tremendous benefit has been realized with the availability of e-mail. "Telephone tag," or repeated phone calls back and forth between callers, has been greatly reduced as messages can be transmitted and retrieved at any hour.

Listserves, or electronic mailing lists, offer web communication with the ability to read and respond to questions and answers, as well as exchange general information with individuals of a common interest. Enrolling to be a part of a listserve insures that information is forwarded to a designated e-mail account on a regular basis. Links are also valuable tools to bring common information to the reader. They are present in many web sites to link the researcher to additional material.

The American Occupational Therapy Association offers listserves and links for specialty areas of interest and practice. Benefits as promoted by AOTA 2000 are reported to be the ability to:

- Share information

- Obtain suggestions for challenging problems

- Find resource information

- Network, and learn about current topics in specialty areas

Subscription is free to AOTA members at www.aota.org and topics of Special Interest Sections (SIS) include:

1. Administration and management

2. Developmental disabilities

3. Education

4. Faculty

5. Fieldwork

6. Research

7. Gerontology

8. Home/community health

9. Mental health

10. Physical disabilities

11. Sensory integration

12. School system

13. Technology

14. Work programs

On-line courses, workshops, or research material makes education in today's world much easier to access. Limitless possibilities exist for information retrieval via the Internet. Internet libraries are available for searching data and providing journal articles and books on most reference topics. University and public libraries across the country, as well as AOTA, allow information retrieval on-line, however there are some charges and membership fees to advance the operations allowed on line. Medline access is available free through PubMed, National Library of Medicine, at www.ncbi.nlm. nih.gov/PubMed/.

Universities, colleges, technical schools, and many professional organizations (including AOTA) offer on-line courses for credit or continuing education units. This method of learning has become extremely popular, especially for rural communities, and distance learning is increasing the ease of access to advanced degrees.

Computer Assisted Evaluation and Treatment Tools

Since the late 1980s, the number of products for computer-assisted evaluations has consistently grown, and new devices continue to be developed. Objective findings have been substantiated with computerized analysis and outcomes management. As technology continues to advance, the occupational therapy manager should welcome these devices that save time, improve productivity, and measure outcomes.

Evaluation

Many products are available for evaluation, including but not limited to: grip and pinch strength collection; hand, upper extremity, and whole body assessment; functional capacity evaluation and work simulation; functional abilities; driving; and home health care. Digital and video cameras can be used for pre- and post-treatment measurements and job site evaluations.

Work Performance Programs

Many work performance models today are using equipment that provides computer-generated reports, outcome measurement, and consumer performance data collection. These systems may utilize exercise baselines and compare data to past as well as normative performance. Depending on equipment used, reports can be generated and findings about performance objectified. See Figure 9.1 for a list of vendors including some work performance equipment.

Treatment Techniques

Assistive technology, assistive devices, hand function, prosthetics, and work performance are some of the primary uses of computer technology at the present time. As advances in electronics and technology are made in the near future, many more options are expected in the area of computerized treatment techniques.

Switches, touch windows, and voice activated word processing programs enable individuals with special needs to operate appliances, computers, keyboards, and mobility devices. In addition to adaptive equipment for daily living skills, there are a significant number of products available for the adult with environmental modification needs. Computer software programs also exist for the cognitive, vocational, and leisure requirements of the individual. Visual perceptual intervention and visual motor processing can also be addressed through the use of such programs.

Hedman (1990, p.3) cautions the therapist and user "not every problem needs a high-tech solution and those that do usually have a low-tech aspect to them." The solution should possess the following attributes:

- Solves the problem
- Does not create additional problems

- Is obtainable by the consumer
- Will be durable in the environment used
- Is serviceable
- Meets the consumers needs

Because there are abundant resources available to the consumer and therapist, Hedman recommends starting with a commercially available item to address the need. Modification of a commercial item is the next step in meeting the consumer need for assistive technology. Finally, custom fabrication of a device can be utilized if step one and two are unsuccessful.

Funding for Technology

An issue critical to occupational therapists regarding technology assistive devices is, "how is it funded?" The occupational therapist is often in a position to request funding. Technology based assistive living devices, as well as other types of adaptive equipment, can be funded by community agencies in some situations. County and state organizations may have funds allotted and/or have received grant monies for families and/or individuals with special needs. Sample letters of justification for a power wheelchair (w/c), positioning equipment, and devices to increase function as provided to a community agency for funding are found in Figures 9.2 and 9.3.

Resources for Assistive Technology

Numerous books and articles have been published and courses designed to guide the user and provider in the use of assistive technology in occupational therapy. On-line websites are readily available. The reader is directed to the list of vendors, including some specific to assistive technology, found in Figure 9.1. In addition, the organizations below may be beneficial for further information, publications, products, and continuing education opportunities regarding assistive technology.

1. Closing the Gap is an organization that focuses on computer technology for people with special needs. A bimonthly newsletter is available as well as an annual international conference and an extensive web site. Visit www.closingthegap.com for links to databases with over 2,000 items.

2. Rehabilitation Engineering and Assistive Technology Society of North America (RESNA) is an interdisciplinary association of people with a common interest in technology and disability. The purpose of RESNA is to promote the potential of people with disabilities through technology, research, development, education, advocacy, and the provision of technology by supporting the people engaged in these activities.

   RESNA programs include the annual conference and exhibit, a journal and other publications, a credentialing program for assistive technology service providers, professional development opportunities, and participation in special interest groups and professional specialty groups.

   Their website offers links to other references as well. To contact RESNA: 1700 N. Moore St., Suite 1540, Arlingon, VA 22209-1903, ph: 703-524-6686, FAX #703-524-6630, TTY 703-524-6639, E-mail – info@resna.org, website www.resna.org.

LETTER OF MEDICAL NECESSITY

MARY

DOB: 3/25/77

DIAGNOSIS: Cerebral palsy, severe cognitive deficits

EQUIPMENT REQUESTED: Metalcraft Modular Seating System with headrest, lap tray and adjustment to current wheelchair including foot plates, calf strap

Mary is a 21 year old female who is completely nonambulatory. She is currently completing her last year in special education at her resident school district. There are plans for her to go to a specialized workshop next year. It is essential that Mary be properly positioned in her wheelchair for her to achieve her maximal potential in these settings.

Current seating components are old and worn. The back can no longer be adjusted properly causing Mary to lean backward with head back and visual attention is generally toward the ceiling. Subsequently she does not readily attend to what is directly in front of her. This will be a disadvantage toward any vocational training. Her seat does not provide adequate support and she slides forward frequently. Recommended modular seating will provide contours in both back and seat components that will provide the stability that Mary needs for optimal function.

Mary also requires that foot plates be replaced. Current foot plates do not fit the wheelchair. She will also require a calf strap to prevent legs from slipping off backwards.

Mary will also require a lap tray for her wheelchair, which will serve as both an upper extremity support and functional work surface.

Thank you for providing this necessary equipment.

_____   _____
Therapist   Date

Figure 9.2. Letter of Justification for Wheelchair Positioning (w/c) *Courtesy of Jeanne Plunkett*

LETTER OF MEDICAL NECESSITY

GEORGE

DOB: 1/18/43

DIAGNOSIS: Degenerative joint disease, obesity, left AKA, CHF

EQUIPMENT REQUESTED: custom oversize power wheelchair with pressure relief cushion and adjustable height armrests, oversize bedside commode

George is a 55 year old male who weighs 425 lbs. He has been a lower extremity amputee for over 30 years and suffers from painful arthritis in all joints but particularly the right knee and left shoulder. He also has a history of bilateral carpal tunnel syndrome and problems with the left rotator cuff. Moving his own weight causes much wear and tear on his joints. He also has cardiac problems. Generally he is able to transfer independently but can have flair ups of arthritic pain so severe that he struggles tremendously. He is able to perform much of his self care, light housekeeping tasks, and is an artist. Goals at this time would be to maintain function as possible through joint preservation, regular activity and range of motion exercises.

A power wheelchair is strongly recommended to accomplish the above goals. Pt will require customization to accommodate his size. The ideal wheelchair will be adjustable to allow for optimal positioning. George requires some back angle recline. Adjustable height armrests are necessary to provide upper extremity support to reduce the destructive effects of inflammation and to provide best leverage for transfer. He will also require a custom seat cushion for pressure relief as he has had incidence of skin breakdown around the coccyx from sitting.

George will also require a bedside commode to use when acute exacerbation of arthritic pain and stiffness greatly hinder his mobility.

Thank you for providing this necessary equipment.

_____   _____
Therapist   Date

Figure 9.3. Letter of Justification for Power Wheelchair (w/c) *Courtesy of Jeanne Plunkett*

3. The American Occupational Therapy Association web page www.aota. org offers a vast array of resources for the occupational therapist. The technology special interest section offers information on products and resources. Using the key words assistive technology services and assistance when searching on the Internet will provide the reader with an abundance of valuable links in this area.

The AOTA offers a "fax on request" line that is helpful to retrieve documents, papers, and many resources via fax. It can be easily accessed by calling 1-800-701-7735. A list of items available can then be faxed using this 24-hour number. Also, of value to the OT manager is the "AOTA Buyer's Guide," published annually in the *OT Practice*.

Other professional associations and organizations hold a wealth of resources for the OT manager. Links from their web addresses to other sources widen the expanse of information. See Figure 9.4 for list of national associations of interest to OT.

Summary

The use of technology for evaluation, treatment, documentation, education, and office management is a tremendous benefit for the OT and manager today. By utilizing the many opportunities available, time and money can be saved while offering greater benefit to the consumer.

Continued advances are expected with a wealth of resources to be promoted for use by individuals with special needs and therapists who service them. Those with spinal cord injuries, and the world continue to hope for technology of miraculous proportions someday. Whatever the future holds for occupational therapists and their consumers, it is likely to provide greater opportunities for independence and function.

Case Study 1

A 16-year old high school student is having difficulty obtaining books, papers, and school supplies independently. Presently these materials are stored in a backpack at the back of the wheelchair.

Discussion Questions

1. What vendors are available that would provide options for the assistive technology needs of this student?
2. Find or create a product to solve the problem.
3. Write a justification letter for funding by a community agency for the item chosen, including cost and specifics of item.

Organization Name	Address	Telephone	Facsimile	E-mail address
American Academy of Orthotists and Prosthetists	1650 King Street, Suite 500 Alexandria, VA 22314	(703) 836-7118	(703) 836-0838	aaopise@aol.com
American Academy of Pain Management	13947 Mono Way, Suite A Sonora, CA 95370	(209) 533-9744	(209) 533-9250	aapm@aol.com
American Academy of Physical Medicine and Rehabilitation	Ore IBM Plaza Chicago, IL 60611-3604	(312) 464-9700	(312) 464-0227	aapmil@aol.com
American Association of Cardiovascular and Pulmonary Rehabilitation	7611 Elmwood Avenue, Suite 201 Middleton, WI 53562	(608) 831-6989	(608) 831-5122	aacpr@imchg.com
American Association of Electrodiagnostic Medicine	21 Second Street SW, Suite 103 Rochester, MN 55902	(507) 288-0100	(507) 288-1225	aaem@aol.com
American Association of Orthopaedic Medicine	435 N. Michigan Avenue, Suite 1717 Chicago, IL 60611-4067	(800) 992-2063	(312) 644-8557	n/a
American Association of Spinal Cord Injury Nurses	75-20 Astoria Blvd. Jackson Heights, NY 11370-1177	(718) 803-3783	(718) 863-0414	n/a
American Board of Physical Medicine and Rehabilitation	21 First Street, SW, Norwest Center, Suite 674 Rochester, MN 55902	(507) 282-1776	(507) 282-9242	n/a
American Chiropractic Association Council on Sports Injuries and Physical Fitness	49 Old Solomons Island Road, Suite 303 Annopolis, MD 21401	(800) 593-3222	(410) 266-8124	n/a
American College of Sports Medicine	401 West Michigan Street Indianapolis, IN 46202-3233	(317) 637-9200	(317) 834-7817	n/a
American Congress of Rehabilitation Medicine	4700 W. Lake Avenue Glenview, IL 60025	(847) 375-4725	(847) 875-4777	n/a
American Physical Therapy Association	1101 17th Street, NW, Suite 1000 Washington, DC 20036	(202) 457-1115	(202) 457-5191	apta@interramp.com
American Occupational Therapy Association	4620 Montgomery Lane, PO Box 31220 Bethesda, MD 20824-1220	(301) 652-2612	(301) 652-7711	n/a
American Rehabilitation Association	1910 Association Drive, 2nd Floor Reston, VA 22091	(703) 648-9300	(703) 648-0346	102262.14@rampaserve.com
American Speech-Language-Hearing Association	10801 Rockville Pike Rockville, MD 20852	(301) 897-5700	(301) 897-7848	n/a
American Spinal Injury Association	345 E. Superior Street, Room 1436 Chicago, IL 60611	(312) 908-6237	(312) 503-0869	n/a
American Subacute Care Association	1440 Kennedy Causeway, Suite 421 North Bay Village, FL 33141	(305) 864-0396	(305) 868-0905	ascamail@aol.com
American Therapeutic Recreation Association	PO Box 15215 Hattiesburg, MS 39404-5215	(800) 553-0304	(800) 264-3337	n/a
Association of Hospital Health and Fitness	915 Elmwood Avenue Evanston, IL 60202	(847) 475-2332	(847) 475-2112	102707.321@compuserve.com
Association of Rehabilitation Nurses	4700 W. Lake Avenue Glenview, IL 60025-1485	(800) 229-7593	(847) 375-4777	arn@anclec.com
Brain Injury Association	1776 Massachusetts Avenue, NW, Suite 100 Washington, DC 20036	(202) 296-6443	(202) 296-8850	n/a
CARF... The Rehabilitation Accreditation Commission	4891 E. Grant Road Tucson, AZ 85712	(520) 325-1044	(520) 318-1129	n/a
Case Management Association of America	8201 Canrell Road, Suite 230 Little Rock, AR 72227	(501) 225-2229	(501) 221-9068	cmsonl@aol.com
Human Factors and Ergonomics Society	PO Box 1369 Santa Monica, CA 93406-1369	(310) 394-1811	(310) 394-2410	72133.1474@compuserve.com
International Association for the Study of Pain	909 NE 43rd Street, Suite 306 Seattle, WA 98105-6020	(206) 547-6409	(206) 547-1703	iasp@locke.hs.washington
The International Functional Electrical Stimulation Society	5030 N. Hill Street Lo Cañada Flintridge, CA 91011	(818) 362-5958	(818) 952-2664	n/a
National Association for Medical Equipment Services	625 Slaters Lane, Suite 200 Alexandria, VA 22314-1171	(703) 836-6263	(703) 836-6730	info@names.org
National Association of Children's Hospitals and Related Institutions	401 Wythe Street Alexandria, VA 22314	(703) 684-1355	(703) 684-1589	n/a
National Association of Orthopaedic Nurses	East Holly Avenue, Box 56 Pitman, NJ 08071-0056	(609) 256-2310	(609) 589-7463	n/a
National Assocation of Rehabilitation Professional in the Private Sector	313 Washington Street, #302 Newton, MA 02158	(617) 558-5333	(617) 692-2040	n/a
National Association of Service Providers in Private Rehabilitation	633 S. Washington Street Alexandria, VA 22314	(206) 523-4964	(206) 526-7194	n/a
National Association of Rehabilitation Agencies	11250 Roger Bacon Drive, Suite B Reston, VA 22090	(703) 437-4377	(703) 435-4390	n/a
National Association for the Support of Long Term Care	4214 Medical Parkway, Suite 209 Austin, TX 78756	(512) 451-8059	(512) 458-3933	n/a
National Athletic Trainers' Association	2952 Stermans Freeway Dallas, TX 75247	(214) 637-6282	(214) 637-2206	webmaster@noto
National Registry of Rehabilitation Technology Suppliers	3223 South Loop 289, Suite 600 Lubbock, TX 79423	(806) 797-7299	(806) 797-8420	n/a
National Spinal Cord Injury Association	545 Concord Avenue, Suite 29 Cambride, MA 2138	(617) 441-8500	(617) 441-3449	nscia@aol.com
North American Society of Gait and Clinical Movement Analysis	200 E. University Avenue St. Paul, MN 55101	(612) 229-3843	(612) 229-3844	gagex091@mo.arin.edu
Paralyzed Veterans of America	801 Eighteenth Street NW Washington, DC 20006	(800) 424-8200	(202) 416-7641	n/a
RESNA	1700 North Moore Street, Suite 540 Arlinton, VA 22209-1903	(703) 524-6684	(703) 524-6630	mailoffics@r

Figure 9.4. List of National Associations

Case Study 2

A private occupational therapy clinic needs to begin submitting their billing electronically to expedite reimbursement.

Discussion Questions

1. Find a medical billing software program that is under $5,000 and is capable of electronic claims submission.
2. Which clearinghouse will be used?
3. Is this clearinghouse able to submit claims to Blue Cross and Blue Shield, Medicare, and Medicaid?
4. What does the clearinghouse charge per claim submitted?

Occupational Therapy Roles

This document is a guide to major roles common in the profession of occupational therapy. It is intended to assist the practitioner in identifying career options and developing career paths. "Practitioner" refers to anyone who is certified by the American Occupational Therapy Certification Board (AOTCB) as an occupational therapist (OTR) or an occupational therapy assistant (COTA). Practitioners work in a variety of systems including health care, educational, academic, governmental, social, corporate, and industrial settings. This document can be a resource for planning career ladders, developing job descriptions, and suggesting educational content for formal and continuing education programs.

Roles listed in this document are those frequently held by certified practitioners and are not all inclusive. The nature of the experience as an occupational therapy practitioner prepares individuals for other specialized roles (e.g., activity director, case manager, rehabilitation coordinator, dean). Roles described in this document are valued equally. Although different roles may vary in their scope and in the experience required to perform them, each role fulfills a specific function within the profession and contributes to the profession's growth, development and strength.

An individual's employment setting, method of service delivery, performance competence, and career goals are all interdependent and result in an individualized composite of roles during actual job performance. In this document, roles are not exclusive because jobs performed by practitioners may include aspects of more than one role. For example, an occupational therapist may have a job that includes practitioner and fieldwork educator roles. Another individual may function as a faculty member, researcher, and consultant.

Career progression involves advancement within roles as well as transition to different roles. When transitioning occurs, practitioners need to have demonstrated performance potential and appropriate educational preparation for the new role. Individuals entering into a new role typically require closer supervision and will begin at a relatively lower level of expertise than in their other roles. Preparation for new roles often involves self-reflection, continuing or advanced education, and acquisition of experience and skills required for the new role. The development of a mentoring relationship assists in understanding the context in which role performance will occur. For example, an individual who is an advanced-level administrator in a practice setting may move into an entry-level faculty role in an academic setting. Preparation for this transition may include acquiring appropriate academic degrees; understanding the educational environment; and demonstrating potential for teaching, scholarly activity, and professional service.

Role Descriptions

Each role in this document consists of the following components: major function, scope of role, performance areas, qualifications, and supervision. These components are described as follows:

Source: Crist, P., Halom, J., Hinjosa, J., McPhee, S., Mitchell, M., Boyt Schell, B., Youngstrom, M.J., Harsh, C. (1993). Occupational Therapy Roles. American Journal of Occupational Therapy, 47(11), 1087–1099.

LEVEL	MAJOR FOCI	SUPERVISION
Entry	• The development of skills. • Socialization in the expectations related to the organization, peers, and the profession. Acceptance of responsibilities and accountability in role relevant professional activities is expected.	Close
Intermediate	• Increased independence. • Mastery of basic role functions. • Ability to respond to situations based on previous experience. • Participation in the education of personnel. Specialization is frequently initiated, along with increased responsibility for collaboration with other disciplines and related organizations. Participation in role-relevant professional activities is increased.	Routine or General
Advanced	• Refinement of specialized skills. • Understanding of complex issues affecting role functions. Contribution to the knowledge base and growth of the profession results in being seen as an expert, resource person, or consultant within a role. This expertise is recognized by others within and outside the profession through leadership, mentoring, research, education, and volunteerism.	Minimal

Table 1   Levels of Role Performance

Major function: Describes the primary purpose(s) of the role.

Scope of role: Delineates the range of responsibility and complexity that typically occurs within the **role.**

Key performance areas: Specifies common activities and expectations associated with role function. Performance that occurs within each area is built upon the unique philosophy and perspective of occupational therapy. Practitioners are expected to take personal responsibility for functioning within the ethical code and standards of the profession. Specific knowledge, skills, and attitudes fundamental for performance are beyond the scope of this document.

Individuals develop varying degrees of expertise in role performance. Levels of expertise are those skills that are fundamental to the entry level, those skills that are intermediate, or those skills that require a high degree of proficiency. These three levels describe the professional development process for each role and are described in Table 1. Progression within a role through the three levels of professional development is based on accumulation of higher level skills through experience, education, guided self-development, and professional socialization. Progression is not simply the amount of time in a role. Each person progresses along this continuum at an individualized pace. Some individuals may remain at one level for the duration of their career and not everyone progress to the advanced level. An individual may function in more than one role simultaneously. When this occurs, it is possible to function at different levels within each role. For example, a new faculty member may be at an entry level in teaching, though at an advanced level in clinical practice. All roles described in this document build on the performance expectations of the Practitioner—OTR and Practitioner—COTA, as this is the entry point into the profession. Consequently, the entry-level performance areas are considered to be an inherent part of all other roles described in this document.

TYPE	DESCRIPTION
Close	Daily, direct contact at the site of work.
Routine	Direct contact at least every 2 weeks at the site of work, with interim supervision occurring by other methods such as telephone or written communication.
General	At least monthly direct contact, with supervision available as needed by other methods.
Minimal	Provided only on a need basis, and may be less than monthly.

Table 2   Levels of Formal Supervision

Supervision: Describes the typical oversight required or recommended for individuals at the various levels of role performance. The amount of supervision required is closely linked to both the role and the level of expertise in a role. The supervision recommended is intended to be a collaborative relationship that serves to promote quality service and the professional development of the individuals involved. All COTAs will require more than a minimal level of supervision by an OTR when providing services. Formal supervision occurs along a continuum including close, routine, general, and minimal. refer to Table 2 for descriptions of these levels.

In addition to formal supervision, individuals may provide or receive functional supervision. Functional supervision implies the provision of information and feedback to coworkers. Individuals who provide functional supervision have specialized knowledge as a result of their own experience and expertise. On the basis of this specialized knowledge or skill, the individual supervises peers relative to this expertise in a particular function. For example, a fieldwork educator may provide functional supervision to coworkers who are supervising students, although he or she is not responsible for evaluating the overall performance of the other therapists.

Qualifications: Lists the critical credentials, education, and work experience necessary as a prerequisite to adequate role performance. Qualifications are listed in a range to reflect changing expectations associated with higher levels of role functioning. As all roles are within the profession, professional certification as a practitioner is a consistent requirement. Additionally, all practitioners are expected to meet state and federal regulatory mandates, adhere to relevant Association policies, and participate in continuing professional development.

Practitioner—OTR

Major Function
Provide quality occupational therapy services, including assessment, intervention, program planning and implementation, discharge planning-related documentation, and communication. Service provision may include direct, monitored, and consultative approaches.

Scope of Role
OTR practitioners advance along a continuum from entry to advanced level based on experience, education, and practice skills. The OTR has the ultimate responsibility for service provision (AOTA, 1990, p.1093).

Key performance areas

Entry-level skills
- Responds to requests for service and initiates referrals when appropriate
- Screens individuals to determine the need for intervention.

- Evaluates individuals to obtain and interpret data necessary for planning intervention and for intervention.
- Interprets evaluation findings to appropriate individuals.
- Develops and coordinates intervention plans, including goals and methods to achieve stated goals.
- Implements the intervention plan directly or in collaboration with others.
- Adapts environment, tools, materials, and activities according to the needs of the individual and his or her social cultural context.
- Monitors the individual's response to intervention and modifies plan as needed.
- Communicates and collaborates with other team members, individuals, family members, or caregivers.
- Follows policies and procedures required in the setting.
- Develops appropriate home and community programming to support performance in natural environment.
- Terminates services when maximum benefit is received and formulates discontinuation and followup plans.
- Documents services as required.
- Maintains records required by practice setting, third-party payers, and regulatory agencies.
- Performs continuous quality improvement activities and program evaluation using predetermined criteria.
- Provides inservice education to team members and the community.
- Maintains treatment area, equipment, and supply inventory.
- Identifies and pursues own professional growth and development.
- Schedules and prioritizes own workload.
- Participates in professional and community activities.
- Monitors own performance and identifies supervisory needs.
- Functions according to the AOTA Code of Ethics (AOTA, 1988) and Standards of Practice (AOTA, 1992) of the profession.

Intermediate skills

- Supervises/teaches occupational therapy practitioners, students, and other staff performing supportive services and/or other aspects of service provision.
- Assists other practitioners in the development of professional skills.
- Participates in committees and activities of larger systems in the development of service operations, policies, and procedures.
- Participates in the fieldwork education process.
- Critically examines own practice and integrates new knowledge.

High-proficiency skills

- Performs advanced, specialized evaluations or interventions.
- Develops protocols and procedures for intervention programs based on current occupational therapy theory and practice.
- Provides expert consultation to practitioners and outside groups about area of expertise.

Qualifications

- Certified by the American Occupational Therapy Certification Board (AOTCB) as an OTR.
- Meets state regulatory requirements.

- Progressive levels of expertise will require one or more of the following: work experience, self-study, continuing education, special certification, or postprofessional education.

Supervision

Practice supervision must be performed by an experienced OTR. Administrative supervision is determined by individual settings and may or may not be performed by an OTR.

- Entry-Level Practitioners—OTRs in a particular practice area will require close supervision for service delivery aspects and routine supervision for administrative aspects (AOTA, 1981).
- Intermediate Practitioners—OTRs require routine to general supervision from advanced practitioners.
- Advanced Practitioners—OTRs require minimal supervision within area of expertise and general supervision for administrative aspects.

Practitioner - COTA

Major Function

Provides quality occupational therapy services to assigned individuals under the supervision of an OTR.

Scope of Role

COTA practitioners advance along a continuum from entry to advanced level, based on experience, education, and practice skills. Development along this continuum is dependent on the development of service competency. The OTR has ultimate overall responsibility for service provision (AOTA, 1990, p.1093).

Key Performance Areas

Entry-level skills

- Responds to request for services in accordance with service agency's policies and procedures.
- Assists with data collection and evaluation under the supervision of an OTR.
- Develops treatment goals under the supervision of an OTR.
- Implements and coordinates intervention plan under the supervision of an OTR.
- Provides direct service that follows a documented routine and accepted procedure under the supervision of an OTR.
- Adapts intervention environment, tools, materials, and activities according to the needs of the individual and his or her sociocultural context under the supervision of an OTR.
- Communicates and interacts with other team members and the individual's family or caregivers in collaboration with an OTR.
- Monitors own performance and identifies supervisory needs.
- Follows policies and procedures required in a setting.
- Performs continuous quality improvement activities or program evaluation in collaboration with an OTR.
- Maintains treatment area, equipment, and supply inventory as required.
- Identifies and pursues own professional growth and development.
- Maintains records and documentation required by work settings under the supervision of an OTR.
- Participates in professional and community activities.
- Functions according to the AOTA Code of Ethics (AOTA, 1988) and Standards of Practice (AOTA, 1992) of the profession.

Intermediate skills

- Schedules and prioritizes own workload.
- Supervises volunteers, COTAs, OTA students, and paersonnel other than OT practitioners under the direction of an OTR.
- Participates in development of policies and procedures in collaboration with an OTR.
- Participates in the fieldwork education process under the direction of an OTR.
- Selects, adapts, and implements intervention under the supervision of an OTR.
- Administers standardized tests under the supervision of an OTR after service competency has been established.
- Modifies treatment approaches to reflect changing needs under the supervision of an OTR.
- Formulates discontinuation and follow-up plans under the supervision of an OTR.
- Participates in organizational activities and committees.

High-proficiency skills

- Serves as a resource person to the agency in areas of specific expertise.
- Educates others in the area of established service competency under the supervision of an OTR.
- Contributes to program planning and development in collaboration with an OTR.

Qualifications:

- Certification by the AOTCB as a COTA.
- Meets state regulatory requirements.
- Progressive levels of expertise will require one or more of the following: work experience, self-study, continuing education, and formal education including advanced degrees.

Supervision

COTAs at all levels require at least general supervision by an OTR. The level of supervision is related to the ability of the COTA to safely and effectively provide those interventions delegated by an OTR. Typically, entry-level COTAs and COTAs new to a particular practice environment will require close supervision, intermediate-level practitioners routine supervision, and advanced-level practitioners general supervision. COTAs will require closer supervision for interventions that are more complex or evaluative in nature and for areas in which service competencies have not been developed. Service competency is the ability to use the identified intervention in a safe and effective manner.

Educator (Consumer, Peer)

Major Function

Develops and provides educational offerings or training related to occupational therapy to consumer, peer, and community individuals or groups.

Scope of Role

Practitioners advance along a continuum of providing informal education to individuals and small groups in the course of service provision, to developing and providing comprehensive educational programs targeted to consumers and peers. At entry level of role, education typically occurs with peers and consumers within the individual's own service system (e.g., patient education, department, or school district inservice). At higher levels of expertise, provision of educational offerings may involve individuals or groups from multiple systems (e.g., provision of injury-prevention programs to industry, caregiver education programs to community, and continuing education seminars).

Performance Areas

Entry-level skills

- Implements strategies to assist individual learner to identify own learning needs.
- Develops or collaborates with individual learner in developing learning objectives.
- Implements educational methods designed to support learner's objectives.
- Responds to feedback about the teaching-learning process, and modifies own educational strategies to support learning.
- Supports the evaluation of educational effectiveness.
- Monitors own performance and identifies own development needs.
- Functions according to the AOTA Code of Ethics (AOTA, 1988) and Standards of Practice (AOTA, 1992) of the profession.

Intermediate skills

- Selects or designs strategies to identify individual learner needs.
- Develops program plans and materials for formal program offerings (e.g., conference presentations, workshops, seminars).
- Uses a variety of teaching-learning methods appropriate to the learning objectives and learner needs.

High-proficiency skills

- Evaluates strategies to identify learning needs of individuals and groups.
- Develops program plans and educational methods for extended or multiple program offerings.
- Designs evaluation strategies to assess impact of educational programs.

Qualifications

- Certification by AOTCB as an OTR or a COTA.
- Progressive levels of expertise will require combinations of the following: self-study, continuing education, experience, and post-entry-level formal education.
- Appropriate level of practice or service expertise is necessary as it relates to provision of these education services.

Supervision

Supervision depends on the nature of the project and the skills of the educator. COTAs at all levels usually will require OTR supervision for educational activities that occur related to occupational therapy consumers.

Fieldwork Educator (Practice Setting)

Major Function

Manages Level I or II fieldwork in a practice setting. Provides occupational therapy or occupational therapy assistant students with opportunities to practice and carry out practitioner competencies.

Scope of Role

The fieldwork educator role may range from supervision of an individual student to full responsibility for an entire fieldwork program.

Key Performance Areas

Entry-level skills

- Establishes, mediates, and supports relationships between practice-based and academic personnel.
- Initiates and maintains communication and correspondence between the practice and academic settings.
- Schedules students in collaboration with the academic fieldwork coordinator.
- Provides orientation for student to fieldwork site including policies, procedures, and student responsibilities.
- Facilitates student learning activities to achieve desired student competence.
- Facilitates student's clinical reasoning and reflective practice.
- Evaluates student performance throughout fieldwork.
- Provides the student with both formative and cumulative feedback and supervision.
- Ensures student's integration of professional standards and ethics into practice.
- Ensures students' compliance with agencies' standards, goals, and objectives.
- Attends meetings, programs, or continuing education related to fieldwork education.
- Develops learning objectives for fieldwork in collaboration with academic institution(s) and consistent with current student fieldwork evaluation(s).
- Functions according to the AOTA Code of Ethics (AOTA, 1988) and Standards of Practice (AOTA, 1992) of the profession.

Intermediate skills

- Provides functional supervision to OTRs and COTAs specific to their roles as student fieldwork supervisors.
- Facilitates assignment of students to appropriate practitioners for supervision.
- Counsels or arbitrates students' concerns.
- Oversees the administrative aspects of the fieldwork program, including the formal agreement with academic programs.
- Conducts ongoing fieldwork program evaluations and monitors changes in program.
- Organizes or participates in appropriate fieldwork education support groups (e.g., local fieldwork councils, Commission on Education).
- Coordinates continuing education and inservice opportunities to develop staff fieldwork education skills.

High-proficiency skills

- Participates at leadership level in appropriate fieldwork groups.
- Facilitates the development of clinical fieldwork programs and related student supervision skills.
- Contributes to student learning by modeling leadership in professional organizations and facilitating student involvement.

Qualifications

- Certified by AOTCB as an OTR or a COTA.

- Meets appropriate state regulatory requirements.
- Continuing education regarding fieldwork education and supervision.
- Entry-level OTRs and COTAs may supervise level I fieldwork students.
- OTRs with 1 year of practice-based experience may supervise OT and OTA Level II fieldwork students.
- COTAs with 1 year of practice-based experience may supervise OTA Level II fieldwork students.
- Three years of experience are recommended for individuals overseeing programs involving multiple student supervisors and multiple students.

Supervision

Supervision provided by an administrator or specifically designated individual. Level of supervision varies with skills of educator, complexity of setting, and nature of student's learning needs.

Supervisor

Major Function(s)

Manages the overall daily operation of occupational therapy services in a defined practice area(s).

Scope of Role

The supervisor is involved in managing other occupational therapy practitioners, personnel, and volunteers in a defined practice setting or program.

Key Performance Areas

Entry-level skills

- Assists in selection, orientation, and training of staff, students, and volunteers.
- Promotes professional growth through staff development.
- Coordinates scheduling of work assignments.
- Evaluates, monitors, and provides feedback regarding job performance of assigned staff.
- Assists in establishment, implementation, and evaluation of agency goals and objectives.
- Monitors and facilitates staff compliance with established standards and guidelines.
- Provides for acquisition, care, and maintenance of physical facilities, supplies, and equipment.
- Oversees implementation of continuous quality improvement activities.
- Represents personnel, fiscal, professional, and program needs to occupational therapy administrator.
- Functions according to the AOTA Code of Ethics (AOTA, 1988) and Standards of Practice (AOTA, 1992) of the profession.

Intermediate skills

- Develops, implements, and monitors department policies and procedures in collaboration with occupational therapy administrator.
- Coordinates specific activities for department or service unit.
- Facilitates collaboration among occupational therapy and non-occupational therapy personnel and administrators.

High-proficiency skills

- Serves as liaison to specialty program coordinators and administrators.

Qualifications

- Certified by AOTCB as an OTR or COTA.
- Meets appropriate state regulatory requirements.
- Two to 3 years of practice experience in service area prior to supervising others are recommended.
- One year of experience is recommended prior to supervising a COTA. Experienced COTAs may supervise other COTAs administratively, as long as service protocols and documentation are supervised by an OTR.
- Continuing or post professional education relevant to supervisory function.

Supervision

Routine to minimal supervision provided by the occupational therapy administrator. Supervision ranges from routine to minimal, depending on the experience and expertise of the supervisor. Consultation from more advanced practitioners should be available as needed.

Administrator (Practice Setting)

Major Function

Manages department, program, services, or agency providing occupational therapy services.

Scope of Role

This role encompasses those individuals who organize and manage occupational therapy service units.

Key Performance Areas

Entry-level skills

- Plans, develops, and monitors occupational therapy services to ensure quality service.
- Achieves service unit goals and objectives through allocation of resources.
- Recruits and hires employees.
- Conducts performance evaluation and staff development activities.
- Establishes policies and standard operating procedures.
- Formulates and manages budget.
- Maintains effective information management systems.
- Assures safe work environments, procedures, and methods.
- Develops and monitors reimbursement processes to support services.
- Monitors the acquisition and maintenance of supplies, equipment, and facilities.
- Develops and supervises a continuous quality improvement program.
- Ensures compliance with accreditation, certification, and government standards.
- Advocates for appropriate use of occupational therapy services.
- Oversees fieldwork education process.
- Functions acccording to the AOTA Code of Ethics (AOTA, 1988) and Standards of Practice (AOTA, 1992) of the profession.

Intermediate skills

- Establishes a long-range plan for staff recruitment, development, and retention.

- Collaborates with other administrators within the organization to develop and manage organizational systems.
- Collaborates with others outside of the organization regarding pertinent administrative management issues.
- Participates at a leadership level in professional, community organizations.

High-proficiency skills

- Participates in organizational strategic planning and establishes strategic plan for assigned areas.
- Develops and implements marketing strategies for assigned areas.
- Facilitates development of systems supporting clinical research.
- Assumes leadership role within the organization and in interorganizational projects.

Qualifications

- Certification by AOTCB as an OTR.
- Meets appropriate state regulatory requirements.
- Graduate degree or continuing education relevant to management.
- Recommended experience varies with size and scope of department; a minimum of 3 years experience is preferred for small programs and 5 or more years for larger programs.

Supervision

General supervision by administrative personnel within the organization is required. Individuals with fewer than 3 years of experience should have access to an occupational therapy management consultant. Consultation from more advanced practitioners should be available as needed.

Consultant

Major Function

Provides occupational therapy consultation to individuals, groups, or organizations.

Scope of Role

Consultative services may take place within the case, colleague, or systems model. Consultation may relate to practice, education, administration, or research.

Key performance Areas

Entry-level skills

- Communicates scope of professional expertise.
- Assists consumers in identifying problems to be addressed in the consultative process.
- Collaborates with consumers in developing appropriate consultation outcomes.
- Develops recommendations that are relevant within the cultural context of the consumers' environment.
- Assists consumers in developing and implementing interventions, or identifying alternate resources necessary to obtain consumer objectives.
- Complies with applicable local, state, and federal laws and regulations.
- Functions according to the AOTA Code of Ethics (AOTA, 1988) and Standards of Practice (AOTA, 1992) of the profession.

Intermediate skills

- Assesses quality of own consultative efforts, and identifies own continuing professional development needs.

High-proficiency skills

- Participates at a leadership level in professional, community organizations.

Qualifications

- Certified by AOTCB as an OTR or COTA.
- Meets appropriate state regulatory requirements.
- Intermediate or advanced practice level.
- Recommend minimum of 6 months experience for case consultation, 1 year for colleague consultation, and 3 to 5 years for systems consultation.

Supervision

Practitioners are expected to function as consultants within the scope of practice appropriate to their level of competence. The OTR functioning as a consultant is responsible for obtaining supervision when needed to meet regulatory and professional standards. The COTA functioning as a consultant is expected to seek the appropriate level of OTR supervision to meet regulatory and professional standards.

Fieldwork Coordinator (Academic Setting)

Major Function

Manages student fieldwork program within the academic setting.

Scope of Role

The fieldwork coordinator role may be decentralized among the faculty or may be managed entirely by one individual. This encompasses all fieldwork experiences required by a curriculum.

Key Performance Areas

Entry-level skills

- Identifies and secures sites for fieldwork education.
- Reviews the quality and appropriateness of fieldwork sites in collaboration with other academic faculty.
- Develops fieldwork objectives in collaboration with the fieldwork sites.
- Initiates and maintains communication and correspondence between the academic and fieldwork sites.
- Communicates with fieldwork educators regarding the curriculum model, course content, and fieldwork expectations.
- Oversees the administrative aspects of the fieldwork program including agreements with fieldwork sites.
- Assigns students to fieldwork settings.
- Orients students to responsibilities and protocol for fieldwork.
- Maintains communication with fieldwork educators and students during fieldwork.
- Monitors the facilitation of clinical reasoning and reflective practice in Level II fieldwork settings.

- Counsels and arbitrates with students and fieldwork educators on matters of concern.
- Collaborates with the fieldwork educator in assigning the final appraisal (grading) of the student.
- Supports research.
- Functions according to the AOTA Code of Ethics (AOTA, 1988) and Standards of Practice (AOTA, 1992) of the profession.
- Participates in appropriate fieldwork educational support groups (e.g., local fieldwork councils, commission on Education).

Intermediate skills

- Provides educational opportunities to prepare and enhance fieldwork educators' knowledge and skills.
- Coordinates continuing education pertaining to fieldwork education processes for clinical fieldwork educators.
- Participates actively in professional, volunteer organizations.
- Supervises support personnel carrying out administrative aspects of fieldwork.

High-proficiency skills

- Participates at leadership level in appropriate fieldwork group.
- Facilitates the development of fieldwork programs and related student supervision skills.

Qualifications

- Certified by AOTCB as an OTR or COTA.
- Three years of practice experience and experience in supervising and advising fieldwork students are recommended.

Supervision

General supervision by academic administrator who is usually the program director. Close to routine supervision for new faculty.

Faculty

Major Function

Provides formal academic education for occupational therapy or occupational therapy assistant students.

Scope of Role

This role varies among institutions and the subsequent balance expected between teaching, service, and scholarly activities. Progression within this role typically advances from lecturer and instructor to the professorial ranks, including assistant, associate, full, and emeritus professorships. Included in the faculty role may be adjunct, clinical, or academic appointments.

Key Performance Areas

Entry-level skills

- Develops educational course objectives and sequences the content to promote optimal learning.
- Designs and structures effective educational experiences, including methods, media, content areas, and types of student interactions.

- Facilitates students' learning through lectures, discussions, practical and laboratory exercises, or practice-related experiences.
- Evaluates and addresses student learning needs within their social and cultural environmental context.
- Reviews educational media and published resources and selects class readings or supplemental materials.
- Plans and prepares course materials to include course syllabi, lectures, case studies, teaching/learning handouts, and questions for group discussion.
- Prepares evaluation materials and measures student attainment of stated course objectives.
- Develops and maintains proficiency in teaching areas through investigation, formal education, continuing education, or practice.
- Participates in curriculum development.
- Participates in teaching evaluation and uses outcome data to modify teaching.
- Advises students and student groups.
- Serves on department, school, college, or university committees.
- Assists with designated departmental administrative tasks such as student admissions, recruitment, and course scheduling.
- Maintains students' records according to regulations and procedures.
- Functions according to AOTA Code of Ethics (AOTA, 1988) and Standards of Practice of (AOTA, 1992) the profession.
- Engages in service to the university or community.

Intermediate skills

- Prepares innovative curriculum or instructional methods.
- Evaluates and incorporates emerging research findings and technology into teaching and research.
- Participates in research and scholarly activities.
- Collaborates in the preparation of academic reports and accreditation self-studies.
- Participates actively in professional organizations.

High-proficiency skills

- Provides expert consultation to practitioners, educators, and outside groups about area of expertise.
- Chairs or leads groups or organizations outside the department.
- Mentors students through scholarly investigation process to develop student skills in research.
- Mentors other faculty in the development of their teaching, research, and practice skills.

Qualifications

- Certified by AOTCB as an OTR or COTA.
- For OTR, in professional programs, a doctoral degree is preferred (a master's degree is recommended).
- In technical programs, a master's degree is preferred (a bachelor's degree is recommended).
- Intermediate to advanced skills in primary area of teaching.
- Skills as a classroom instructor and understanding of the educational system.

Supervision

General supervision by academic program director and other appropriate academic administrators. Close to routine supervision by academic program directors for new, adjunct, and part-time faculty.

Program Director (Academic Setting)

Major Function

Manages the occupational therapy educational program.

Scope of Role

The program director's role varies depending on the level of the program (e.g., technical, professional, or post-professional level) and the demands of the academic setting (e.g., technical school, community college, college, university, or health sciences center). The academic program director facilitates the education of competent graduates through faculty development and supervision and effective program management. Dependent on their academic environment, program directors may oversee both academic and practice-related activities, externally funded projects, and continuing education programs.

Key Performance Areas

Entry-level skills

- Oversees student recruitment, selection, evaluation, advisement, retention, and professional development.
- Oversees institutional and professional accreditation activities and reports.
- manages faculty recruitment, development, evaluation, and retention.
- Assigns and monitors faculty and staff responsibilities.
- Ensures the quality of the program.
- Formulates and implements a fiscal plan.
- Represents the program to university administrators and negotiates for the needs of the program.
- Fosters an academic climate that facilitates faculty, student, and staff learning and professional growth.
- Promotes effective instructional techniques for faculty.
- Oversees student and faculty rights and responsibilities.
- Produces narrative and data-based reports for internal and external communication.
- Facilitates library acquisitions of resources for teaching and research.
- Fosters beneficial relationships among faculty and practitioners.
- Functions according to the AOTA Code of Ethics (AOTA, 1988) and Standards of Practice (AOTA, 1992) of the profession.

Intermediate skills

- Develops and implements long-range or strategic plans.
- Produces scholarly work.
- Facilitates the development of useful information management systems.
- Participates at the leadership level in professional and community organizations.

High-proficiency skills

- Leads in the acquisition of externally funded projects.
- Designs and implements marketing for program enhancement.
- Promotes central theme within the occupational therapy programs that contribute to the knowledge base of the profession.

Qualifications

Technical-Level Program Director

- An OTR with a bachelor's degree (a master's degree is preferred) who is certified by AOTCB.
- Recommend 3 years professional practice with experience supervising COTAs.
- Recommend 3 years experience as a faculty member.
- Experience or continuing education in academic management.

Professional-Level Program Director

- An OTR with a master'd degree (a doctoral degree is preferred) who is certified by AOTCB.
- Recommend 5 years experience in practice.
- Recommend 5 years experience as a faculty member.
- Experience or continuing education in academic management.

Post-Professional-Level Program Director

- An OTR with a doctoral degree who is certified by AOTCB
- Recommended 5 years experience in practice.
- Recommended 5 years experience as a faculty member.
- Experience or continuing education in academic management.
- Intermediate to advanced competence as a researcher/scholar.

Supervision

General to minimal administrative supervision from designated administrative officer. Individuals with fewer than 3 years experience should have access to occupational therapy education and accreditation consultants.

Researcher/Scholar

Major Function

Performs scholarly work of the profession including examining, developing, refining, and evaluating the profession's body of knowledge, theoretical base, and philosophical foundations.

Scope of Role

The role of the researcher ranges from the individual who critically examines and interprets empirical studies to independent investigator. The scholar is an individual who has in-depth knowledge and who engages in examination, development, or refinement of the profession's body of knowledge.

Key Performance Areas:

Entry-level skills

- Promotes and engages in research/scholarly activities.

- Reads, interprets, and applies scholarly information relative to occupational therapy.
- Collects research data.
- Assumes responsibility for the ethical concerns in research and complies with institutional bio-ethics committee protocols.
- Functions according to the AOTA Code of Ethics (AOTA, 1988) and the Standards of Practice (AOTA, 1992) of the profession.

Intermediate skills

- Directs the completion of studies, including data analysis, interpretation, and dissemination of results.
- Collaborates with others to facilitate studies of concern to the profession.
- Monitors resources which facilitate research and scholarly activities.

High-proficiency skills

- Probes methods of science, theoretical information, or research designs to answer questions important to the profession.
- Conceptualizes the body of knowledge in the profession to develop new theories, frames of reference, or models of practice.
- Mentors novice researchers.
- Participates at the leadership level in professional, volunteer organizations.

Qualifications

- Certified by AOTCB as an OTR or COTA.
- Progressive levels of expertise will require combinations of the following: self-study, continuing education, experience, and formal education for independent research or scholarly activitites.
- COTAs can contribute to the research process. COTAs need additional academic qualifications to be a principal investigator.

Supervision

Supervision ranges from close to minimal, depending on the nature of the project and the skills of the researcher/scholar.

Entrepreneur

Major Function

Entrepreneurs are partially or fully self-employed individuals who provide occupational therapy services.

Scope of Role

Entrepreneurs may function in a variety of roles, including independent contractor and private practice owner or operator. The form of organization may be sole proprietorship, partnership, corporation, group practice, or joint venture.

Key Performance Areas

Entry-level skills

- Delivers quality occupational therapy services within scope of endeavor.

- Develops and implements business plan designed to ensure viability using financial and legal consultation.
- Establishes a business organization appropriate to nature and scope of activities.
- Negotiates contractual relationships that take into account the setting, services, and reimbursement.
- Uses legal, financial, and practice consultation as needed to support business operations.
- Establishes and collects fees for service, complying with reimbursement requirements.
- Manages business support services.
- Complies with local, state, and federal laws and regulations related to business and practice.
- Complies with standards and guidelines of accrediting or regulating organizations.
- Develops and maintains personnel policies and records.
- Develops and implements marketing strategies, as appropriate.
- Evaluates consumer satisfaction and business operations.
- Develops and implements risk management plan that includes business property, liability, and employee or employer benefits.
- Functions according to the AOTA Code of Ethics (AOTA, 1988) and Standards of Practice (AOTA, 1992) of the profession, as well as business ethics.

Intermediate skills
- Participates in, supervises, or oversees fieldwork program.
- Participates at a leadership level in professional, community organizations.

Qualifications
- Certified by AOTCB as an OTR or COTA.
- Meets appropriate state regulatory requirements.
- A minimum of 3 years of practice experience.

Supervision
In cases in which a COTA provides direct service, it is the COTA's responsibility to obtain the appropriate level of supervision from an OTR. Expert consultation or mentorship is obtained as needed to support the business. legal, financial, regulatory, and practice aspects of role performance.

References

American Occupational Therapy Association. (1981). Guide to supervision of occupational therapy personnel. *American Journal of Occupational Therapy, 35,* 815-816.

American Occupational Therapy Association. (1988). Occupational therapy code of ethics. *American Journal of Occupational Therapy, 42,* 795-796

American Occupational Therapy Association. (1990). Entry-level role delineation for registered occupational therapists (OTRs) and certified occupational therapy assistants (COTAs). *American Journal of Occupational Therapy, 44,* 1091-1102.

American Occupational Therapy Association, (1992). Standards of practice. *American Journal of Occupational Therapy, 46,* 1082-1085.

Related Background Materials

American Occupational Therapy Association. (1991). Essentials and guidelines for an accredited educational program for the occupational therapist. *American Journal of Occupational Therapy, 45,* 1077-1084.

American Occupational Therapy Association. (1991). Essentials and guidelines for an accredited education program for the occupational therapy assistant. *American Journal of Occupational Therapy, 45,* 1085-1092.

American Occupational Therapy Association. (in press). Guide to supervision of occupational therapy personnel. (1988). In *Reference manual of official documents of The American Occupational Therapy Association, Inc.* Rockville, MD: Author. (Original work published 1981, *American Journal of Occupational Therapy, 35,* 815-816.)

Beeler, J. L, Young, P. A. & Dull, S. M. (1990). Professional development framework: Pathway to the future. *Journal of Nursing Staff Development, 6,* 296-301.

Mitchell, M.M. (1985). Professional development: Clinician to academician. *American Journal of Occupational Therapy, 39,* 368-373.

Appendix

The need for a broader description of career options for occupational therapy was identified as part of the Entry-Level Study Report (AOTA, 1987) presented t the Representative Assembly (RA). The RA charged the Executive Board to study the recommendation of the Entry-Level Report and develop an action plan. The Executive Board formed a Directions for the Future (DFF) Coordinating Committee and charged that committee to develop an overall action plan. part of the action plan was the implementation of a DFF Symposium to examine the future needs of practice and education.

Following the symposium, the DFF Coordinating Committee directed the Commission on Education (COE) and Commission on Practice (COP) to form a combined task force of members to develop a document describing a hierarchy of occupational therapy roles. The chairpersons of both commissions selected representatives from a wide variety of arenas in both practice and education. The task force included individuals directly involved in both professional and technical levels of education and practice. Special Interest Section Steering Committee (SISSC) representation was added to the task force to further broaden the scope of the task force. Reference to current professional literature provided a foundation for committee work. The most important references are listed at the end of this section.

Throughout the entire document development process, the document was reviewed by the members of the full COE, COP, COTA Task Force, and SISSC, as well as program directors for professional and technical curricula, thus ensuring both OTR and COTA perspectives. One preliminary review of this document was followed by two formal reviews of drafts. The commission chairpersons recommended that the task force report be sent to the Intercommission Council (ICC) to further ensure that all facets of the Association were represented in the document development process.

As a result of the task force and review processes, an integrated education and practice taxonomy was recommended by the task force rather than a hierarchy. The taxonomy was preferred because it would provide practical information for a variety of uses within the profession. Since this taxonomy is a classification of categories of professional roles, it was decided to entitle the document Occupational Therapy Roles.

An ad hoc task force representing the Commission on Education Steering Committee (COESC), the Commission on Practice (COP), and the Special Interest Sections Steering Committee (SISSC) met in 1991 to 1992 and developed this draft entitled, Occupational Therapy Roles. This document is expected to replace and expand on the Guide to Classification of Occupational Therapy Personnel (AOTA, 1987).

Reference

American Occupational Therapy Association. (1987). Guide to classification of occupational therapy personnel. In *Reference manual of official documents of The American Occupational Therapy Association, Inc.* Rockville, MD: Author. (Original work published 1985, American Journal of Occupational Therapy, 39, 803-810.

Standards of Practice for Occupational Therapy

Preface

The *Standards of Practice for Occupational Therapy* are requirements for the occupational therapy practitioner (registered occupational therapist and certified occupational therapy assistant) for the delivery of occupational therapy services that are client centered and interactive in nature (American Occupational Therapy Association [AOTA], 1995). The registered occupational therapist supervises the certified occupational therapy assistant, and both work together in a collaborative manner to meet the needs of the client. However, the registered occupational therapist is ultimately responsible and accountable for the delivery of occupational therapy services. This document identifies minimum standards for occupational therapy practice.

The minimum educational requirements for the registered occupational therapist are described in the current *Essentials and Guidelines of an Accredited Educational Program for the Occupational Therapist* (AOTA, 1991a). The minimum educational requirements for the certified occupational therapy assistant are described in the current *Essentials and Guidelines of an Accredited Educational Program for the Occupational Therapy Assistant* (AOTA, 1991b).

Definitions

Assessment. Specific tools, instruments, or interactions used during the evaluation process. An assessment is a component part of the evaluation process (Hinojosa & Kramer, 1998).

Client. A person, group, program, organization, or community for whom the occupational therapy practitioner is providing services (AOTA, 1995).

Evaluation. The process of obtaining and interpreting data necessary for understanding the individual, system, or situation. This includes planning for and documenting the evaluation process, results, and recommendations, including the need for intervention and/or potential change in the intervention plan (Hinojosa & Kramer, 1998).

Source:
   Author: Commission on Practice, Linda Kohlman Thomson, MOT, OT(C), FAOTA, Chairperson
   Adopted by the Representative Assembly 1998M15 NOTE: This document replaces the 1994 Standards of Practice for Occupational Therapy.

Occupational therapy practitioner. Any individual initially certified to practice as an occupational therapist or occupational therapy assistant or licensed or regulated by a state, district, commonwealth, or territory of the United States to practice as an occupational therapist or occupational therapy assistant (AOTA, 1997).

Performance areas: Broad categories of human activity that are typically part of daily life. They are activities of daily living, work and productive activities, and play or leisure activities (AOTA, 1994c).

Performance components. Elements of performance required for successful engagement in performance areas, including sensorimotor, cognitive, psychosocial, and psychological aspects (AOTA, 1994c).

Performance contexts. Situations or factors that influence an individual's engagement in desired and/or required performance areas. Performance contexts consist of temporal aspects (chronological, developmental, life cycle, disability status) and environmental aspects (physical, social, political, cultural) (AOTA, 1994c).

Screening. Obtaining and reviewing data relevant to a potential client to determine the need for further evaluation and intervention.

Transition. Process involving actions coordinated to prepare for or facilitate change, such as from one functional level to another, from one life stage to another, from one program to another, or from one environment to another.

Standard I: Professional Standing and Responsibility

1. An occupational therapy practitioner delivers occupational therapy services that reflect the philosophical base of occupational therapy (AOTA, 1979) and are consistent with the established principles and concepts of theory and practice.

2. An occupational therapy practitioner delivers occupational therapy services in accordance with AOTA's standards and policies. The nature and scope of occupational therapy services provided must be in accordance with laws and regulations.

3. An occupational therapy practitioner maintains current licensure, registration, or certification as required by laws or regulations.

4. An occupational therapy practitioner abides by AOTA's Occupational Therapy Code of Ethics (AOTA, 1994a).

5. An occupational therapy practitioner assures continued competency by establishing, maintaining, and updating professional performance, knowledge, and skills.

6. A registered occupational therapist provides supervision for a certified occupational therapy assistant in a collaborative manner as defined by official AOTA documents and in accordance with laws or regulations.

7. A certified occupational therapy assistant seeks and follows supervision from a registered occupational therapist in the delivery of occupational therapy services.

8. An occupational therapy practitioner is knowledgeable about AOTA's Standards of Practice for Occupational Therapy; the Philosophical Base of Occupational Therapy (AOTA, 1979); and other AOTA, state, and federal documents relevant to practice and service delivery.

9. An occupational therapy practitioner maintains current knowledge of legislative, political, social, cultural, and reimbursement issues that affect clients and the practice of occupational therapy.

10. A registered occupational therapist is knowledgeable about research in the practitioner's areas of practice. A registered occupational therapist applies timely research findings ethically and appropriately to evaluation and intervention processes and discusses applicable research findings with the certified occupational therapy assistant.

11. A registered occupational therapist systematically assesses the efficiency and effectiveness of occupational therapy services and designs and implements processes to support quality service delivery.

12. A certified occupational therapy assistant collaborates with the registered occupational therapist in assessing the efficiency and effectiveness of occupational therapy services and assists in designing and implementing processes to support quality service delivery.

Standard II: Referral

1. A registered occupational therapist accepts and responds to referrals in accordance with AOTA's Statement of Occupational Therapy Referral (AOTA, 1994b) and in compliance with laws or regulations.

2. A registered occupational therapist accepts and responds to referrals for evaluation or evaluation with intervention in performance areas, performance components, or performance contexts when clients may have a functional limitation or disability or may be at risk for a disabling condition.

3. A registered occupational therapist refers clients to appropriate resources when the needs of the client can best be served by the expertise of other professionals or services.

4. An occupational therapy practitioner educates current and potential referral sources about the scope of occupational therapy services and the process of initiating occupational therapy services.

Standard III: Screening

1. A registered occupational therapist screens independently or as a member of a team in accordance with laws and regulations. A certified occupational therapy assistant may contribute to the screening process under the supervision of a registered occupational therapist.

2. A registered occupational therapist selects screening methods appropriate to the client's performance context.

3. A registered occupational therapist communicates screening results and recommendations to the appropriate person, group, or organization. A certified occupational therapy assistant may contribute to this process under the supervision of a registered occupational therapist.

Standard IV: Evaluation

1. A registered occupational therapist evaluates performance areas, performance components, and performance contexts. A certified occupational therapy assistant may contribute to the evaluation process under the supervision of a registered occupational therapist.

2. An occupational therapy practitioner educates clients and appropriate others about the purposes and procedures of the occupational therapy evaluation.

3. A registered occupational therapist selects assessments to evaluate the client's level of function related to performance areas, performance components, and performance contexts.

4. An occupational therapy practitioner follows defined protocols when standardized assessments are used.

5. A registered occupational therapist analyzes, interprets, and summarizes assessment data to determine the client's current functional status and to develop an appropriate intervention plan. The certified occupational therapy assistant may contribute to this process under the supervision of a registered occupational therapist.

6. A registered occupational therapist completes and documents occupational therapy evaluation results within the time frames, formats, and standards established by practice settings,

government agencies, external accreditation programs, and payers. A certified occupational therapy assistant may contribute to documentation of evaluation results under the supervision of a registered occupational therapist and in accordance with laws or regulations.

7. A registered occupational therapist communicates evaluation results, within the boundaries of client confidentiality, to the appropriate person, group, or organization. A certified occupational therapy assistant may contribute to this process under the supervision of a registered occupational therapist.

8. A registered occupational therapist recommends additional consultations when the results of the evaluation indicate that intervention by other professionals would be beneficial.

Standard V: Intervention Plan

1. A registered occupational therapist develops and documents an intervention plan that is based on the results of the occupational therapy evaluation and the desires and expectations of the client and appropriate others about the outcome of service. A certified occupational therapy assistant may contribute to the intervention plan under the supervision of a registered occupational therapist.

2. A registered occupational therapist ensures that the intervention plan is documented within time frames, formats, and standards established by the practice settings, agencies, external accreditation programs, and payers.

3. A registered occupational therapist includes in the intervention plan client-centered goals that are clear, measurable, behavioral, functional, contextually relevant, and appropriate to the client's needs, desires, and expected outcomes. A certified occupational therapy assistant may contribute to this process.

4. A registered occupational therapist includes in the intervention plan the scope, frequency, duration of services, and the needs of the client.

5. A registered occupational therapist reviews the intervention plan with the client and appropriate others. A certified occupational therapy assistant may contribute to this process.

Standard VI: Intervention

1. A registered occupational therapist implements the intervention plan through the use of specified purposeful activities or therapeutic methods that are meaningful to the client and are effective methods for enhancing occupational performance. A certified occupational therapy assistant may implement the intervention plan under the supervision of a registered occupational therapist.

2. An occupational therapy practitioner informs clients and appropriate others regarding the relative benefits and risks of the intervention.

3. An occupational therapy practitioner maintains or seeks current information on resources relevant to the client's needs.

4. A registered occupational therapist reevaluates during the intervention process and documents changes in the client's goals, performance, and needs. A certified occupational therapy assistant may contribute to the reevaluation process.

5. A registered occupational therapist modifies the intervention process to reflect changes in client status, desires, and response to intervention. A certified occupational therapy assistant may identify the need for modifications and may contribute to the intervention modifications under the supervision of a registered occupational therapist.

6. An occupational therapy practitioner documents the occupational therapy services provided within the time frames, formats, and standards established by the practice settings, agencies, external accreditation programs, and payers.

Standard VII: Transition Services

1. A registered occupational therapist prepares a formal transition plan that is based on identified needs. A certified occupational therapy assistant may contribute to the preparation of a formal transition plan.

2. An occupational therapy practitioner facilitates the transition process in cooperation with the client, family members, significant others, team, and community resources and individuals, when appropriate.

Standard VIII: Discontinuation

1. A registered occupational therapist discontinues services when the client has achieved predetermined goals, has achieved maximum benefit from occupational therapy services, or does not desire to continue services. A certified occupational therapy assistant may recommend discontinuation of occupational therapy services to the supervising registered occupational therapist.

2. A registered occupational therapist prepares and implements a discontinuation plan that addresses appropriate follow-up resources. A certified occupational therapy assistant may contribute to the implementation of a discontinuation plan under the supervision of a registered occupational therapist.

3. A registered occupational therapist documents changes in the client's status between the initial evaluation and discontinuation of services. A certified occupational therapy assistant may contribute to the process under the supervision of a registered occupational therapist.

4. A registered occupational therapist documents recommendations for follow-up or reevaluation, when applicable.

References

American Occupational Therapy Association (1979). The philosophical base of occupational therapy. *American Journal of Occupational Therapy, 33,* 785.

American Occupational Therapy Association. (1991a). Essentials and guidelines of an accredited educational program for the occupational therapist. *American Journal of Occupational Therapy. 45,* 1077-1084.

American Occupational Therapy Association. (1991b). Essentials and guidelines of an accredited educational program for the occupational therapy assistant. *American Journal of Occupational Therapy, 45,* 1085-1092.

American Occupational Therapy Association. (1994a). Occupational therapy code of ethics. *American Journal of Occupational Therapy, 48,* 1037-1038.

American Occupational Therapy Association. (1994b). Statement of occupational therapy referral. *American Journal of Occupational Therapy, 48,* 1034.

American Occupational Therapy Association. (1994c). Uniform terminology for occupational therapy-Third edition. *American Journal of Occupational Therapy, 49,* 1047-1054.

American Occupational Therapy Association. (1995). Concept paper: Service delivery in occupational therapy. *American Journal of Occupational Therapy, 49,* 1029-1031.

American Occupational Therapy Association. (1997). Bylaws. Article III, Section 1. Bethesda, MD: Author.

Hinojosa, J., & Kramer, P. (Eds.). (1998) *Occupational therapy evaluation of clients: Obtaining and interpreting data.* Bethesda, MD: American Occupational Therapy Association.

Occupational Therapy Code of Ethics—2000

Preamble

The American Occupational Therapy Association's Code of Ethics is a public statement of the common set of values and principles used to promote and maintain high standards of behavior in occupational therapy. The American Occupational Therapy Association and its members are committed to furthering the ability of individuals, groups, and systems to function within their total environment. To this end, occupational therapy personnel (including all staff and personnel who work and assist in providing occupational therapy services, (e.g., aides, orderlies, secretaries, technicians) have a responsibility to provide services to recipients in any stage of health and illness who are individuals, research participants, institutions and businesses, other professionals and colleagues, students, and to the general public.

The *Occupational Therapy Code of Ethics* is a set of principles that applies to occupational therapy personnel at all levels. These principles to which occupational therapists and occupational therapy assistants aspire are part of a lifelong effort to act in an ethical manner. The various roles of practitioner (occupational therapist and occupational therapy assistant), educator, fieldwork educator, clinical supervisor, manager, administrator, consultant, fieldwork coordinator, faculty program director, researcher/scholar, private practice owner, entrepreneur, and student are assumed.

Any action in violation of the spirit and purpose of this Code shall be considered unethical. To ensure compliance with the Code, the Commission on Standards and Ethics (SEC) establishes and maintains the enforcement procedures. Acceptance of membership in the American Occupational Therapy Association commits members to adherence to the code of Ethics and its enforcement procedures. The Code of Ethics, Core Values and Attitudes of Occupational Therapy Practice (AOTA, 1993), and the Guidelines to the Occupational Therapy Code of Ethics (AOTA, 1998) are aspirational documents designed to be used together to guide occupational therapy personnel.

Principal 1. Occupational therapy personnel shall demonstrate a concern for the well-being of the recipients of their services. (beneficence)

Source: AOTA (2000) in The Reference Manual of the Official Document of the American Occupational Therapy Assoc., 115–119, Bethesda. Authors: The Commission on Standards and Ethics (SEC): Barbara L. Kornblau, JD, OTR, FAOTA, Chairperson; Melba Arnold, MS, OTR/L; Nancy Nashiro, PhD, OTR, FAOTA; Diane Hill, COTA/L, AP; Deborah Y. Slater, MS, OTR/L; John Morris, PhD; Linda Withers, CNHA, FACH-CA; Penny Kyler, MA, OTR/L, FAOTA, Staff Liaison. April 2000. Adopted by the Representative Assembly 2000M15. Note: This document replaces the 1994 document, Occupational Therapy Code of Ethics (American Journal of Occupational Therapy, 48, 1037-1038). Prepared 4/7/2000

A. Occupational therapy personnel shall provide services in a fair and equitable manner. They shall recognize and appreciate the cultural components of economics, geography, race, ethnicity, religious and political factors, marital status, sexual orientation, and disability of all recipients of their services.

B. Occupational therapy practitioners shall strive to ensure that fees are fair and reasonable and commensurate with services performed. When occupational therapy practitioners set fees, they shall set fees considering institutional, local, state, and federal requirements, and with due regard for the service recipient's ability to pay.

C. Occupational therapy personnel shall make every effort to advocate for recipients to obtain needed services through available means.

Principle 2. Occupational therapy personnel shall take reasonable precautions to avoid imposing or inflicting harm upon the recipient of services or to his or her property. (nonmaleficence)

A. Occupational therapy personnel shall maintain relationships that do not exploit the recipient of services sexually, physically, emotionally, financially, socially, or in any other manner.

B. Occupational therapy practitioners shall avoid relationships or activities that interfere with professional judgment and objectivity.

Principle 3. Occupational therapy personnel shall respect the recipient and/or their surrogate(s) as well as the recipient's rights. (autonomy, privacy, confidentiality)

A. Occupational therapy practitioners shall collaborate with service recipients or their surrogate(s) in setting goals and priorities throughout the intervention process.

B. Occupational therapy practitioners shall fully inform the service recipients of the nature, risks, and potential outcomes of any interventions.

C. Occupational therapy practitioners shall obtain informed consent from participants involved in research activities and indicate that they have fully informed and advised the participants of potential risks and outcomes. Occupational therapy practitioners shall endeavor to ensure that the participant(s) comprehend these risks and outcomes.

D. Occupational therapy personnel shall respect the individual's right to refuse professional services or involvement in research or educational activities.

E. Occupational therapy personnel shall protect all privileged confidential forms of written, verbal, and electronic communication gained from educational, practice, research, and investigational activities unless otherwise mandated by local, state, or federal regulations.

Principle 4. Occupational therapy personnel shall achieve and continually maintain high standards of competence. (duties)

A. Occupational therapy practitioners shall hold the appropriate national and state credentials for the services they provide.

B. Occupational therapy practitioners shall use procedures that conform to the standards of practice and other appropriate AOTA documents relevant to practice.

C. Occupational therapy practitioners shall take responsibility for maintaining and documenting competence by participating in professional development and educational activities.

D. Occupational therapy practitioners shall critically examine and keep current with emerging knowledge relevant to their practice so they may perform their duties on the basis of accurate information.

E. Occupational therapy practitioners shall protect service recipients by ensuring that duties assumed by or assigned to other occupational therapy personnel match credentials, qualifications, experience, and scope of practice.

F. Occupational therapy practitioners shall provide appropriate supervision to individuals for whom the practitioners have supervisory responsibility in accordance with Association policies, local, state and federal laws, and institutional values.

G. Occupational therapy practitioners shall refer to or consult with other service providers whenever such a referral or consultation would be helpful to the care of the recipient of service. The referral or consultation process should be done in collaboration with the recipient of service.

Principle 5. Occupational therapy personnel shall comply with laws and Association policies guiding the profession of occupational therapy. (justice)

A. Occupational therapy personnel shall familiarize themselves with and seek to understand and abide by applicable Association policies; local, state, and federal laws; and institutional rules.

B. Occupational therapy practitioners shall remain abreast of revisions in those laws and Association policies that apply to the profession of occupational therapy and shall inform employers, employees, and colleagues of those changes.

C. Occupational therapy practitioners shall require those they supervise in occupational therapy-related activities to adhere to the Code of Ethics.

D. Occupational therapy practitioners shall take reasonable steps to ensure employers are aware of occupational therapy's ethical obligations, as set forth in this Code of Ethics, and of the implications of those obligations for occupational therapy practice, education, and research.

E. Occupational therapy practitioners shall record and report in an accurate and timely manner all information related to professional activities.

Principle 6. Occupational therapy personnel shall provide accurate information about occupational therapy services. (veracity)

A. Occupational therapy personnel shall accurately represent their credentials, qualifications, education, experience, training, and competence. This is of particular importance for those to whom occupational therapy personnel provide their services or with whom occupational therapy practitioners have a professional relationship.

B. Occupational therapy personnel shall disclose any professional, personal, financial, business. or volunteer affiliations that may pose a conflict of interest to those with whom they may establish a professional, contractual, or other working relationship.

C. Occupational therapy personnel shall refrain from using or participating in the use of any form of communication that contains false, fraudulent, deceptive, or unfair statements or claims.

D. Occupational therapy practitioners shall accept the responsibility for their professional actions which reduce the public's trust in occupational therapy services and those that perform those services.

Principle 7. Occupational therapy personnel shall treat colleagues and other professionals with fairness, discretion, and integrity. (fidelity)

A. Occupational therapy personnel shall preserve, respect, and safeguard confidential information about colleagues and staff, unless otherwise mandated by national, state, or local laws.

B. Occupational therapy practitioners shall accurately represent the qualifications, views, contributions, and findings of colleagues.

C. Occupational therapy personnel shall take adequate measures to discourage, prevent, expose, and correct any breaches of the Code of Ethics and report any breaches of the Code of Ethics to the appropriate authority.

D. Occupational therapy personnel shall familiarize themselves with established policies and procedures for handling concerns about this Code of Ethics, including familiarity with national, state, local, district, and territorial procedures for handling ethics complaints. These include policies and procedures created by the American Occupational Therapy Association, licensing and regulatory bodies, employers, agencies, certification boards, and other organizations who have jurisdiction over occupational therapy practice.

References

American Occupational Therapy Association. (1993). Core values and attitudes of occupational therapy practice. *American Journal of Occupational Therapy, 47,* 1085-1086.

American Occupational Therapy Association. (1998). Guidelines to the occupational therapy code of ethics. *American Journal of Occupational Therapy, 52,* 881-884.

Americans with Disabilities Act Questions and Answers

Barriers to employment, transportation, public accommodations, public services, and telecommunications have imposed staggering economic and social costs on American society and have undermined our well-intentioned efforts to educate, rehabilitate, and employ individuals with disabilities. By breaking down these barriers, the Americans with Disabilities Act (ADA) will enable society to benefit from the skills and talents of individuals with disabilities, will allow us all to gain from their increased purchasing power and ability to use it, and will lead to fuller, more productive lives for all Americans.

The Americans with Disabilities Act gives civil rights protections to individuals with disabilities similar to those provided to individuals on the basis of race, color, sex, national origin, age, and religion. It guarantees equal opportunity for individuals with disabilities in public accommodations, employment, transportation, State and local government services, and telecommunications.

Fair, swift, and effective enforcement of this landmark civil rights legislation is a high priority of the Federal Government. This booklet is designed to provide answers to some of the most often asked questions about the ADA.

For answers to additional questions, call the ADA Information Line

800-514-0301 (voice)

800-514-0383 (TDD)

Additional ADA resources are listed in the Resources section of this document, page 170.

July 1996

Employment

Q. What employers are covered by title I of the ADA, and when is the coverage effective?

A. The title I employment provisions apply to private employers, State and local governments, employment agencies, and labor unions. Employers with 25 or more employees were covered as of July 26, 1992. Employers with 15 or more employees were covered two years later, beginning July 26, 1994.

Q. What practices and activities are covered by the employment nondiscrimination requirements?

Source: U.S. Equal Employment Opportunity Commission, U.S. Department of Justice Civil Rights Division

A. The ADA prohibits discrimination in all employment practices, including job application procedures, hiring, firing, advancement, compensation, training, and other terms, conditions, and privileges of employment. It applies to recruitment, advertising, tenure, layoff, leave, fringe benefits, and all other employment-related activities.

Q. Who is protected from employment discrimination?

A. Employment discrimination is prohibited against "qualified individuals with disabilities." This includes applicants for employment and employees. An individual is considered to have a "disability" if s/he has a physical or mental impairment that substantially limits one or more major life activities, has a record of such an impairment, or is regarded as having such an impairment. Persons discriminated against because they have a known association or relationship with an individual with a disability also are protected.

The first part of the definition makes clear that the ADA applies to persons who have impairments and that these must substantially limit major life activities such as seeing, hearing, speaking, walking, breathing, performing manual tasks, learning, caring for oneself, and working. An individual with epilepsy, paralysis, HIV infection, AIDS, a substantial hearing or visual impairment, mental retardation, or a specific learning disability is covered, but an individual with a minor, nonchronic condition of short duration, such as a sprain, broken limb, or the flu, generally would not be covered.

The second part of the definition protecting individuals with a record of a disability would cover, for example, a person who has recovered from cancer or mental illness.

The third part of the definition protects individuals who are regarded as having a substantially limiting impairment, even through they may not have such an impairment. For example, this provision would protect a qualified individual with a severe facial disfigurement from being denied employment because an employer feared the "negative reactions" of customers or co-workers.

Q. Who is a "qualified individual with a disability?"

A. A qualified individual with a disability is a person who meets legitimate skill, experience, education, or other requirements of an employment position that s/he holds or seeks, and who can perform the essential functions of the position with or without reasonable accommodation. Requiring the ability to perform "essential" functions assures that an individual with a disability will not be considered unqualified simply because of inability to perform marginal or incidental job functions. If the individual is qualified to perform essential job functions except for limitations caused by a disability, the employer must consider whether the individual could perform these functions with a reasonable accommodation. If a written job description has been prepared in advance of advertising or interviewing applicants for a job, this will be considered as evidence, although not conclusive evidence, of the essential functions of the job.

Q. Does an employer have to give preference to a qualified applicant with a disability over other applicants?

A. No. An employer is free to select the most qualified applicant available and to make decisions based on reasons unrelated to a disability. For example, suppose two persons apply for a job as a typist and an essential function of the job is to type 75 words per minute accurately. One applicant, an individual with a disability, who is provided with a reasonable accommodation for a typing test, types 50 words per minute; the other applicant who has no disability accurately types 75 words per minute. The employer can hire the applicant with the higher typing speed, if typing speed is needed for successful performance of the job.

Q. What limitations does the ADA impose on medical examinations and inquiries about disability?

A. An employer may not ask or require a job applicant to take a medical examination before making a job offer. It cannot make any pre-employment inquiry about a disability or the nature or severity of a disability. An employer may, however, ask questions about the ability to perform specific job functions and may, with certain limitations, ask an individual with a disability to describe or demonstrate how s/he would perform these functions.

An employer may condition a job offer on the satisfactory result of a post-offer medical examination or medical inquiry if this is required of all entering employees in the same job category. A post-offer examination or inquiry does not have to be job-related and consistent with business necessity.

However, if an individual is not hired because a post-offer medical examination or inquiry reveals a disability, the reason(s) for not hiring must be job-related and consistent with business necessity. The employer also must show that no reasonable accommodation was available that would enable the individual to perform the essential job functions, or that accommodation would impose an undue hardship. A post-offer medical examination may disqualify an individual if the employer can demonstrate that the individual would pose a "direct threat" in the workplace (i.e., a significant risk of substantial harm to the health or safety of the individual or others) that cannot be eliminated or reduced below the direct threat level through reasonable accommodation. Such a disqualification is job-related and consistent with business necessity. A post-offer medical examination may not disqualify an individual with a disability who is currently able to perform essential job functions because of speculation that the disability may cause a risk of future injury.

After a person starts work, a medical examination or inquiry of an employee must be job-related and consistent with business necessity. Employers may conduct employee medical examinations where there is evidence of a job performance or safety problem, examinations required by other Federal laws, examinations to determine current fitness to perform a particular job, and voluntary examinations that are part of employee health programs.

Information from all medical examinations and inquiries must be kept apart from general personnel files as a separate, confidential medical record, available only under limited conditions.

Tests for illegal use of drugs are not medical examinations under the ADA and are not subject to the restrictions of such examinations.

Q. When can an employer ask an applicant to "self-identify" as having a disability?

A. Federal contractors and subcontractors who are covered by the affirmative action requirements of section 503 of the Rehabilitation Act of 1973 may invite individuals with disabilities to identify themselves on a job application form or by other pre-employment inquiry, to satisfy the section 503 affirmative action requirements. Employers who request such information must observe section 503 requirements regarding the manner in which such information is requested and used, and the procedures for maintaining such information as a separate, confidential record, apart from regular personnel records.

A pre-employment inquiry about a disability is allowed if required by another Federal law or regulation such as those applicable to disabled veterans and veterans of the Vietnam era. Pre-employment inquiries about disabilities may be necessary under such laws to identify applicants or clients with disabilities in order to provide them with required special services.

Q. Does the ADA require employers to develop written job descriptions?

A. No. The ADA does not require employers to develop or maintain job descriptions. However, a written job description that is prepared before advertising or interviewing applicants for a job will be considered as evidence along with other relevant factors. If an employer uses job descriptions, they should be reviewed to make sure they accurately reflect the actual functions of a job. A job description will be most helpful if it focuses on the results or outcome of a job function, not solely on the way it customarily is performed. A reasonable accommodation may enable a person with a disability to accomplish a job function in a manner that is different from the way an employee who is not disabled may accomplish the same function.

Q. What is "reasonable accommodation?"

A. Reasonable accommodation is any modification or adjustment to a job or the work environment that will enable a qualified applicant or employee with a disability to participate in the application process or to perform essential job functions. Reasonable accommodation also includes adjustments to assure that a qualified individual with a disability has rights and privileges in employment equal to those of employees without disabilities.

Q. What are some of the accommodations applicants and employees may need?

A. Examples of reasonable accommodation include making existing facilities used by employees readily accessible to and usable by an individual with a disability; restructuring a job; modifying work schedules; acquiring or modifying equipment; providing qualified readers or interpreters; or appropriately modifying examinations, training, or other programs. Reasonable accommodation also may include reassigning a current employee to a vacant position for which the individual is qualified, if the person is unable to do the original job because of a disability even with an accommodation. However, there is no obligation to find a position for an applicant who is not qualified for the position sought. Employers are not required to lower quality or quantity standards as an accommodation; nor are they obligated to provide personal use items such as glasses or hearing aids.

The decision as to the appropriate accommodation must be based on the particular facts of each case. In selecting the particular type of reasonable accommodation to provide, the principal test is that of effectiveness, i.e., whether the accommodation will provide an opportunity for a person with a disability to achieve the same level of performance and to enjoy benefits equal to those of an average, similarly situated person without a disability. However, the accommodation does not have to ensure equal results or provide exactly the same benefits.

Q. When is an employer required to make a reasonable accommodation?

A. An employer is only required to accommodate a "known" disability of a qualified applicant or employee. The requirement generally will be triggered by a request from an individual with a disability, who frequently will be able to suggest an appropriate accommodation. Accommodations must be made on an individual basis, because the nature and extent of a disabling condition and the requirements of a job will vary in each case. If the individual does not request an accommodation, the employer is not obligated to provide one except where an individual's known disability impairs his/her ability to know of, or effectively communicate a need for, an accommodation that is obvious to the employer. If a person with a disability requests, but cannot suggest, an appropriate accommodation, the employer and the individual should work together to identify one. There are also many public and private resources that can provide assistance without cost.

Q. What are the limitations on the obligation to make a reasonable accommodation?

A. The individual with a disability requiring the accommodation must be otherwise qualified, and the disability must be known to the employer. In addition, an employer is not required to make an accommodation if it would impose an "undue hardship" on the operation of the employer's business. "Undue hardship" is defined as an "action requiring significant difficulty or expense" when considered in light of a number of factors. These factors include the nature and cost of the accommodation in relation to the size, resources, nature, and structure of the employer's operation. Undue hardship is determined on a case-by-case basis. Where the facility making the accommodation is part of a larger entity, the structure and overall resources of the larger organization would be considered, as well as the financial and administrative relationship of the facility to the larger organization. In general, a larger employer with greater resources would be expected to make accommodations requiring greater effort or expense than would be required of a smaller employer with fewer resources.

If a particular accommodation would be an undue hardship, the employer must try to identify another accommodation that will not pose such a hardship. Also, if the cost of an accommodation would impose an undue hardship on the employer, the individual with a disability should be given the option of paying that portion of the cost which would constitute an undue hardship or providing the accommodation.

Q. Must an employer modify existing facilities to make them accessible?

A. The employer's obligation under title I is to provide access for an individual applicant to participate in the job application process, and for an individual employee with a disability to perform the essential functions of his/her job, including access to a building, to the work site, to needed equipment, and to all facilities used by employees. For example, if an employee lounge is located in a place inaccessible to an employee using a wheelchair, the lounge might be modified or relocated, or comparable facilities might be provided in a location that would enable the individual to take a break with co-workers. The employer must provide such access unless it would cause an undue hardship.

Under title I, an employer is not required to make its existing facilities accessible until a particular applicant or employee with a particular disability needs an accommodation, and then the modifications should meet that individual's work needs. However, employers should consider initiating changes that will provide general accessibility, particularly for job applicants, since it is likely that people with disabilities will be applying for jobs. The employer does not have to make changes to provide access in places or facilities that will not be used by that individual for employment-related activities or benefits.

Q. Can an employer be required to reallocate an essential function of a job to another employee as a reasonable accommodation?

A. No. An employer is not required to reallocate essential functions of a job as a reasonable accommodation.

Q. Can an employer be required to modify, adjust, or make other reasonable accommodations in the way a test is given to a qualified applicant or employee with a disability?

A. Yes. Accommodations may be needed to assure that tests or examinations measure the actual ability of an individual to perform job functions rather than reflect limitations caused by the disability. Tests should be given to people who have sensory, speaking, or manual impairments in a format that does not require the use of the impaired skill, unless it is a job-related skill that the test is designed to measure.

Q. Can an employer maintain existing production/performance standards for an employee with a disability?

A. An employer can hold employees with disabilities to the same standards of production/performance as other similarly situated employees without disabilities for performing essential job functions, with or without reasonable accommodation. An employer also can hold employees with disabilities to the same standards of production/performance as other employees regarding marginal functions unless the disability affects the person's ability to perform those marginal functions. If the ability to perform marginal functions is affected by the disability, the employer must provide some type of reasonable accommodation such as job restructuring but may not exclude an individual with a disability who is satisfactorily performing a job's essential functions.

Q. Can an employer establish specific attendance and leave policies?

A. An employer can establish attendance and leave policies that are uniformly applied to all employees, regardless of disability, but may not refuse leave needed by an employee with a disability if other employees get such leave. An employer also may be required to make adjustments in leave policy as a reasonable accommodation. The employer is not obligated to provide additional paid leave, but accommodations may include leave flexibility and unpaid leave.

A uniformly applied leave policy does not violate the ADA because it has a more severe effect on an individual because of his/her disability. However, if an individual with a disability requests a modification of such a policy as a reasonable accommodation, an employer may be required to provide it, unless it would impose an undue hardship.

Q. Can an employer consider health and safety when deciding whether to hire an applicant or retain an employee with a disability?

A. Yes. The ADA permits employers to establish qualification standards that will exclude individuals who pose a direct threat – i.e., a significant risk of substantial harm – to the health or safety of the individual or of others, if that risk cannot be eliminated or reduced below the level of a direct threat by reasonable accommodation. However, an employer may not simply assume that a threat exists; the employer must establish through objective, medically supportable methods that there is a significant risk that substantial harm could occur in the workplace. By requiring employers to make individualized judgements based on reliable medical or other objective evidence rather than on generalizations, ignorance, fear, patronizing attitudes, or stereotypes, the ADA recognizes the need to balance the interests of people with disabilities against the legitimate interests of employers in maintaining a safe workplace.

Q. Are applicants or employees who are currently illegally using drugs covered by the ADA?

A. No. Individuals who currently engage in the illegal use of drugs are specifically excluded from the definition of a "qualified individual with a disability" protected by the ADA when the employer takes action on the basis of their drug use.

Q. Is testing for the illegal use of drugs permissible under the ADA?

A. Yes. A test for the illegal use of drugs is not considered a medical examination under the ADA; therefore, employers may conduct such testing of applicants or employees and make employment decisions based on the results. The ADA does not encourage, prohibit, or authorize drug tests.

If the results of a drug test reveal the presence of a lawfully prescribed drug or other medical information, such information must be treated as a confidential medical record.

Q. Are alcoholics covered by the ADA?

A. Yes. While a current illegal user of drugs is not protected by the ADA if an employer acts on the basis of such use, a person who currently uses alcohol is not automatically denied protection. An alcoholic is a person with a disability and is protected by the ADA if s/he is qualified to perform the essential functions of the job. An employer may be required to provide an accommodation to an alcoholic. However, an employer can discipline, discharge or deny employment to an alcoholic whose use of alcohol adversely affects job performance or conduct. An employer also may prohibit the use of alcohol in the workplace and can require that employees not be under the influence of alcohol.

Q. Does the ADA override Federal and State health and safety laws?

A. The ADA does not override health and safety requirements established under other Federal laws even if a standard adversely affects the employment of an individual with a disability. If a standard is required by another Federal law, an employer must comply with it and does not have to show that the standard is job related and consistent with business necessity. For example, employers must conform to health and safety requirements of the U.S. Occupational Safety and Health Administration. However, an employer still has the obligation under the ADA to consider whether there is a reasonable accommodation, consistent with the standards of other Federal laws, that will prevent exclusion of qualified individuals with disabilities who can perform jobs without violating the standards of those laws. If an employer can comply with both the ADA and another Federal law, then the employer must do so.

The ADA does not override State or local laws designed to protect public health and safety, except where such laws conflict with the ADA requirements. If there is a State or local law that would exclude an individual with a disability from a particular job or profession because of a health or safety risk, the employer still must assess whether a particular individual would pose a "direct threat" to health or safety under the ADA standard. If such a "direct threat" exists, the employer must consider whether it could be eliminated or reduced below the level of a "direct threat" by reasonable accommodation. An employer cannot rely on a State or local law that conflicts with ADA requirements as a defense to a charge of discrimination.

Q. How does the ADA affect workers' compensation programs?

A. Only injured workers who meet the ADA's definition of an "individual with a disability" will be considered disabled under the ADA, regardless of whether they satisfy criteria for receiving benefits under workers' compensation or other disability laws. A worker also must be "qualified" (with or without reasonable accommodation) to be protected by the ADA. Work-related injuries do not always cause physical or mental impairments severe enough to "substantially limit" a major life activity. Also, many on-the-job injuries cause temporary impairments which heal within a short period of time with little or no long-term or permanent impact. Therefore, many injured workers who qualify for benefits under workers' compensation or other disability benefits laws may not be protected by the ADA. An employer must consider work-related injuries on a case-by-case basis to know if a worker is protected by the ADA.

An employer may not inquire into an applicant's workers' compensation history before making a conditional offer of employment. After making a conditional job offer, an employer may inquire about a person's workers compensation history in a medical inquiry or examination that is required of all applicants in the same job category. However, even after a conditional offer has been made, an employer cannot require a potential employee to have a medical examination because a response to a medical inquiry (as opposed to results from a medical examination) shows a previous on-the-job injury unless all applicants in the same job category are required to have an examination. Also, an employer may not base an employment decision on the speculation that an applicant may cause increased workers' compensation costs in the future. However, an employer may refuse to hire, or may discharge an individual who is not currently able to perform a job without posing a significant risk of substantial harm to the health or safety of the individual or others, if the risk cannot be eliminated or reduced by reasonable accommodation.

An employer may refuse to hire or may fire a person who knowingly provides a false answer to a lawful post-offer inquiry about his/her condition or worker's compensation history.

An employer also may submit medical information and records concerning employees and applicants (obtained after a conditional job offer) to state workers' compensation offices and "second injury" funds without violating ADA confidentiality requirements.

Q. What is discrimination based on "relationship or association" under the ADA?

A. The ADA prohibits discrimination based on relationship or association in order to protect individuals from actions based on unfounded assumptions that their relationship to a person with a disability would affect their job performance, and from actions caused by bias or misinformation concerning certain disabilities. For example, this provision would protect a person whose spouse has a disability from being denied employment because of an employer's unfounded assumption that the applicant would use excessive leave to care for the spouse. It also would protect an individual who does volunteer work for people with AIDS from a discriminatory employment action motivated by that relationship or association.

Q. How are the employment provisions enforced?

A. The employment provisions of the ADA are enforced under the same procedures now applicable to race, color, sex, national origin, and religious discrimination under title VII of the Civil Rights Act of 1964, as amended, and the Civil Rights Act of 1991. Complaints regarding actions that occurred on or after July 26, 1992, may be filed with the Equal Employment Opportunity Commission or designated State human rights agencies. Available remedies will include hiring, reinstatement, promotion, back pay, front pay, restored benefits, reasonable accommodation, attorneys' fees, expert witness fees, and court costs. Compensatory and punitive damages also may be available in cases of intentional discrimination or where an employer fails to make a good faith effort to provide a reasonable accommodation.

Q. What financial assistance is available to employers to help them make reasonable accommodations and comply with the ADA?

A. A special tax credit is available to help smaller employers make accommodations required by the ADA. An eligible small business may take a tax credit of up to $5,000 per year for accommodations made to comply with the ADA. The credit is available for one-half of the cost of "eligible access expenditures" that are more than $250 but less than $10,250.

A full tax deduction, up to $15,000 per year, also is available to any business for expenses of removing qualified architectural or transportation barriers. Expenses covered include costs of removing barriers created by steps, narrow doors, inaccessible parking spaces, restroom facilities, and transportation vehicles. Information about the tax credit and the tax deduction can be obtained from a local IRS office, or by contacting the Office of Chief Counsel, Internal Revenue Service.

Tax credits are available under the Targeted Jobs Tax Credit Program (TJTCP) for employers who hire individuals with disabilities referred by State or local vocational rehabilitation agencies, State Commissions on the Blind, or the U.S. Department of Veterans Affairs, and certified by a State Employment Service. Under the TJTCP, a tax credit may be taken for up to 40 percent of the first $6,000 of a first-year wages of a new employee with a disability. This program must be reauthorized each year by Congress. Further information about the TJTCP can be obtained from the State Employment Services or from State Governors' Committees on the Employment of People with Disabilities.

Q. What are an employer's recordkeeping requirements under the employment provisions of the ADA?

A. An employer must maintain records such as application forms submitted by applicants and other records related to hiring, requests for reasonable accommodation, promotion, demotion, transfer, layoff or termination, rates of pay or other terms of compensation, and selection for training or apprenticeship for one year after making the record or taking the action described (whichever occurs later). If a charge of discrimination is filed or an action is brought by EEOC, an employer must save all personnel records related to the charge until final disposition of the charge.

Q. Does the ADA require that an employer post a notice explaining its requirements?

A. The ADA requires that employers post a notice describing the provisions of the ADA. It must be made accessible, as needed, to individuals with disabilities. A poster is available from EEOC summarizing the requirements of the ADA and other Federal legal requirements for nondiscrimination for which EEOC has enforcement responsibility. EEOC also provides guidance on making this information available in accessible formats for people with disabilities.

Q. What resources does the Equal Employment Opportunity Commission have available to help employers and people with disabilities understand and comply with the employment requirements of the ADA?

A. The Equal Employment Opportunity Commission has developed several resources to help employers and people with disabilities understand and comply with the employment provisions of the ADA.

Resources include:

A Technical Assistance Manual that provides "how-to" guidance on the employment provisions of the ADA as well as a resource directory to help individuals find specific information.

A variety of brochures, booklets, and fact sheets.

For information on how to contact the Equal Employment Opportunity Commission, see page 170.

State and Local Governments

Q. Does the ADA apply to State and local governments?

A. Title II of the ADA prohibits discrimination against qualified individuals with disabilities in all programs, activities, and services of public entities. It applies to all State and local governments, their departments and agencies, and any other instrumentalities or special purpose districts of State or local governments. It clarifies the requirements of section 504 of the Rehabilitation Act of 1973 for public transportation systems that receive Federal financial assistance, and extends coverage to all public entities that provide public transportation, whether or not they receive Federal financial assistance. It establishes detailed standards for the operation of public transit systems, including commuter and intercity rail (AMTRAK).

Q. When do the requirements for State and local governments become effective?

A. In general, they became effective on January 26, 1992.

Q. How does title II affect participation in a State or local government's programs, activities, and services?

A. A state or local government must eliminate any eligibility criteria for participation in programs, activities, and services that screen out or tend to screen out persons with disabilities, unless it can establish that the requirements are necessary for the provision of the service, program, or activity. The State or local government may, however, adopt legitimate safety requirements necessary for safe operation if they are based on real risks, not on stereotypes or generalizations about individuals with disabilities. Finally, a public entity must reasonably modify its policies, practices, or procedures to avoid discrimination. If the public entity can demonstrate that a particular modification would fundamentally alter the nature of its service, program, or activity, it is not required to make that modification.

Q. Does title II cover a public entity's employment policies and practices?

A. Yes. Title II prohibits all public entities, regardless of the size of their work force, from discriminating in employment against qualified individuals with disabilities. In addition to title II's employment coverage, title I of the ADA and section 504 of the Rehabilitation Act of 1973 prohibit employment discrimination against qualified individuals with disabilities by certain public entities.

Q. What changes must a public entity make to its existing facilities to make them accessible?

A. A public entity must ensure that individuals with disabilities are not excluded from services, programs, and activities because existing buildings are inaccessible. A State or local government's programs, when viewed in their entirety, must be readily accessible to and usable by individuals with disabilities. This standard, known as "program accessibility," applies to facilities of a public entity that existed on January 26, 1992. Public entities do not necessarily have to make each of their existing facilities accessible. They may provide program accessibility by a number of methods including alteration of existing facilities, acquisition or construction of additional facilities, relocation of a service or program to an accessible facility, or provision of services at alternate accessible sites.

Q. When must structural changes be made to attain program accessibility?

A. Structural changes needed for program accessibility must be made as expeditiously as possible, but no later than January 26, 1995. This three-year time period is not a grace period; all alterations must be accomplished as expeditiously as possible. A public entity that employs 50 or more persons must have developed a transition plan by July 26, 1992, setting forth the steps necessary to complete such changes.

Q. What is self-evaluation?

A. A self-evaluation is a public entity's assessment of its current policies and practices. The self-evaluation identifies and corrects those policies and practices that are inconsistent with title II's requirements. All public entities must complete a self-evaluation by January 26, 1993. A public entity that employs 50 or more employees must retain its self-evaluation for three years. Other public entities are not required to retain their self-evaluations, but are encouraged to do so because these documents evidence a public entity's good faith efforts to comply with title II's requirements.

Q. What does title II require for new construction and alterations?

A. The ADA requires that all new buildings constructed by a State or local government be accessible. In addition, when a State or local government undertakes alterations to a building, it must make the altered portions accessible.

Q. How will a State or local government know that a new building is accessible?

A. A State or local government will be in compliance with the ADA for new construction and alterations if it follows either of two accessibility standards. It can choose either the Uniform Federal Accessibility Standards or the Americans with Disabilities Act Accessibility Guidelines for Buildings and Facilities, which is the standard that must be used for public accommodations and commercial facilities under title III of the ADA. If the State or local government chooses the ADA Accessibility Guidelines, it is not entitled to the elevator exemption (which permits certain private buildings under three stories or under 3,000 square feet per floor to be constructed without an elevator).

Q. What requirements apply to a public entity's emergency telephone services, such as 911?

A. State and local agencies that provide emergency telephone services must provide "direct access" to individuals who rely on a TDD or computer modem for telephone communication. Telephone access through a third party or through a relay service does not satisfy the requirement for direct access. Where a public entity provides 911 telephone service, it may not substitute a separate seven-digit telephone line as the sole means for access to 911 services by nonvoice users. A public entity may, however, provide a separate seven-digit line for the exclusive use of nonvoice callers in addition to providing direct access for such calls to its 911 line.

Q. Does title II require that telephone emergency service systems be compatible with all formats used for nonvoice communications?

A. No. At present, telephone emergency services must only be compatible with the Baudot format. Until it can be technically proven that communications in another format can operate in a reliable and compatible manner in a given telephone emergency environment, a public entity would not be required to provide direct access to computer modems using formats other than Baudot.

Q. How will the ADA's requirements for State and local governments be enforced?

A. Private individuals may bring lawsuits to enforce their rights under title II and may receive the same remedies as those provided under section 504 of the Rehabilitation Act of 1973, including reasonable attorney's fees. Individuals may also file complaints with eight designated Federal agencies, including the Department of Justice and the Department of Transportation.

Public Accommodations

Q. What are public accommodations?

A. A public accommodation is a private entity that owns, operates, leases, or leases to, a place of public accommodation. Places of public accommodation include a wide range of entities, such as restaurants, hotels, theaters, doctors' offices, pharmacies, retail stores, museums, libraries, parks, private schools, and day care centers. Private clubs and religious organizations are exempt from the ADA's title III requirements for public accommodations.

Q. Will the ADA have any effect on the eligibility criteria used by public accommodations to determine who may receive services?

A. Yes. If a criterion screens out or tends to screen out individuals with disabilities, it may only be used if necessary for the provision of the services. For instance, it would be a violation for a retail store to have a rule excluding all deaf persons from entering the premises, or for a movie theater to exclude all individuals with cerebral palsy. More subtle forms of discrimination are also prohibited. For example, requiring presentation of a driver's license as the sole acceptable means of identification for purposes of paying by check could constitute discrimination against individuals with vision impairments. This would be true if such individuals are ineligible to receive licenses and the use of an alternative means of identification is feasible.

Q. Does the ADA allow public accommodations to take safety factors into consideration in providing services to individuals with disabilities?

A. The ADA expressly provides that a public accommodation may exclude an individual, if that individual poses a direct threat to the health or safety of others that cannot be mitigated by appropriate modifications in the public accommodation's policies or procedures, or by the provision of auxiliary aids. A public accommodation will be permitted to establish objective safety criteria for the operation of its business; however, any safety standard must be based on objective requirements rather than stereotypes or generalizations about the ability of persons with disabilities to participate in an activity.

Q. Are there any limits on the kinds of modifications in policies, practices, and procedures required by the ADA?

A. Yes. The ADA does not require modifications that would fundamentally alter the nature of the services provided by the public accommodation. For example, it would not be discriminatory for a physician specialist who treats only burn patients to refer a deaf individual to another physician for treatment of a broken limb or respiratory ailment. To require a physician to accept patients outside of his or her specialty would fundamentally alter the nature of the medical practice.

Q. What kinds of auxiliary aids and services are required by the ADA to ensure effective communication with individuals with hearing or vision impairments?

A. Appropriate auxiliary aids and services may include services and devices such as qualified interpreters, assistive listening devices, notetakers, and written materials for individuals with hearing impairments; and qualified readers, taped texts, and brailled or large print materials for individuals with vision impairments.

Q. Are there any limitations on the ADA's auxiliary aids requirements?

A. Yes. The ADA does not require the provision of any auxiliary aid that would result in an undue burden or in a fundamental alteration in the nature of the goods or services provided by a public accommodation. However, the public accommodation is not relieved from the duty to furnish an alternative auxiliary aid, if available, that would not result in a fundamental alteration or undue burden. Both of these limitations are derived from existing regulations and caselaw under section 504 of the Rehabilitation Act and are to be determined on a case-by-case basis.

Q. Will restaurants be required to have brailled menus?

A. No, not if waiters or other employees are made available to read the menu to a blind customer.

Q. Will a clothing store be required to have brailled price tags?

A. No, not if sales personnel could provide price information orally upon request.

Q. Will a bookstore be required to maintain a sign language interpreter on its staff in order to communicate with deaf customers?

A. No, not if employees communicate by pen and notepad when necessary.

Q. Are there any limitations on the ADA's barrier removal requirements for existing facilities?

A. Yes. Barrier removal need be accomplished only when it is "readily achievable" to do so.

Q. What does the term "readily achievable" mean?

A. It means "easily accomplishable and able to be carried out without much difficulty or expense."

Q. What are examples of the types of modifications that would be readily achievable in most cases?

A. Examples include the simple ramping of a few steps, the installation of grab bars where only routine reinforcement of the wall is required, the lowering of telephones, and similar modest adjustments.

Q. Will businesses need to rearrange furniture and display racks?

A. Possibly. For example, restaurants may need to rearrange tables and department stores may need to adjust their layout of racks and shelves in order to permit access to wheelchair users.

Q. Will businesses need to install elevators?

A. Businesses are not required to retrofit their facilities to install elevators unless such installation is readily achievable, which is unlikely in most cases.

Q. When barrier removal is not readily achievable, what kinds of alternative steps are required by the ADA?

A. Alternatives may include such measures as in-store assistance for removing articles from inaccessible shelves, home delivery of groceries, or coming to the door to receive or return dry cleaning.

Q. Must alternative steps be taken without regard to cost?

A. No, only readily achievable alternative steps must be undertaken.

Q. How is "readily achievable" determined in a multisite business?

A. In determining whether an action to make a public accommodation accessible would be "readily achievable," the overall size of the parent corporation or entity is only one factor to be considered. The ADA also permits consideration of the financial resources of the particular facility or facilities involved and the administrative or fiscal relationship of the facility or facilities to the parent entity.

Q. Who has responsibility for ADA compliance in leased places of public accommodation, the landlord or the tenant?

A. The ADA places the legal obligation to remove barriers or provide auxiliary aids and services on both the landlord and the tenant. The landlord and the tenant may decide by lease who will actually make the changes and provide the aids and services, but both remain legally responsible.

Q. What does the ADA require in new construction?

A. The ADA requires that all new construction of places of public accommodation, as well as of "commercial facilities" such as office buildings, be accessible. Elevators are generally not required in facilities under three stories or with fewer than 3,000 square feet per floor, unless the building is a shopping center or mall; the professional office of a health care provider; a terminal, depot, or other public transit station; or an airport passenger terminal.

Q. Is it expensive to make all newly constructed places of public accommodation and commercial facilities accessible?

A. The cost of incorporating accessibility features in new construction is less than one percent of construction costs. This is a small price in relation to the economic benefits to be derived from full accessibility in the future, such as increased employment and consumer spending and decreased welfare dependency.

Q. Must every feature of a new facility be accessible?

A. No, only a specified number of elements such as parking spaces and drinking fountains must be made accessible in order for a facility to be "readily accessible." Certain nonoccupiable spaces such as elevator pits, elevator penthouses, and piping or equipment catwalks need not be accessible.

Q. What are the ADA requirements for altering facilities?

A. All alterations that could affect the usability of a facility must be made in an accessible manner to the maximum extent feasible. For example, if during renovations a doorway is being relocated, the new doorway must be wide enough to meet the new construction standard for accessibility. When alterations are made to a primary function area, such as the lobby of a bank or the dining area of a cafeteria, an accessible path of travel to the altered area must also be provided. The bathrooms, telephones, and drinking fountains serving that area must also be made accessible. These additional accessibility alterations are only required to the extent that the added accessibility costs do not exceed 20% of the cost of the original alteration. Elevators are generally not required in facilities under three stories or with fewer than 3,000 square feet per floor, unless the building is a shopping center or mall; the professional office of a health care provider; a terminal, depot, or other public transit station; or an airport passenger terminal.

Q. Does the ADA permit an individual with a disability to sue a business when that individual believes that discrimination is about to occur, or must the individual wait for the discrimination to occur?

A. The ADA public accommodations provisions permit an individual to allege discrimination based on a reasonable belief that discrimination is about to occur. This provision, for example, allows a person who uses a wheelchair to challenge the planned construction of a new place of public accommodation, such as a shopping mall, that would not be accessible to individuals who use wheelchairs. The resolution of such challenges prior to the construction of an inaccessible facility would enable any necessary remedial measures to be incorporated in the building at the planning stage, when such changes would be relatively inexpensive.

Q. How does the ADA affect existing State and local building codes?

A. Existing codes remain in effect. The ADA allows the Attorney General to certify that a State law, local building code, or similar ordinance that establishes accessibility requirements meets or exceeds the minimum accessibility requirements for public accommodations and commercial facilities. Any State or local government may apply for certification of its code or ordinance. The Attorney General can certify a code or ordinance only after prior notice and a public hearing at which interested people, including individuals with disabilities, are provided an opportunity to testify against the certification.

Q. What is the effect of certification of a State or local code or ordinance?

A. Certification can be advantageous if an entity has constructed or altered a facility according to a certified code or ordinance. If someone later brings an enforcement proceeding against the entity, the certification is considered "rebuttable evidence" that the State law or local ordinance meets or exceeds the minimum requirements of the ADA. In other words, the entity can argue that the construction or alteration met the requirements of the ADA because it was done in compliance with the State or local code that had been certified.

Q. When are the public accommodations provisions effective?

A. In general, they became effective on January 26, 1992.

Q. How will the public accommodations provisions be enforced?

A. Private individuals may bring lawsuits in which they can obtain court orders to stop discrimination. Individuals may also file complaints with the Attorney General, who is authorized to bring lawsuits in cases of general public importance or where a pattern or practice of discrimination is alleged. In these cases, the Attorney General may seek monetary damages and civil penalties. Civil penalties may not exceed $50,000 for a first violation or $100,000 for any subsequent violation.

Miscellaneous

Q. Is the Federal government covered by the ADA?

A. The ADA does not cover the executive branch of the Federal government. The executive branch continues to be covered by title V of the Rehabilitation Act of 1973, which prohibits discrimination in services and employment on the basis of handicap and which is a model for the requirements of the ADA. The ADA, however, does cover Congress and other entities in the legislative branch of the Federal government.

Q. Does the ADA cover private apartments and private homes?

A. The ADA does not cover strictly residential private apartments and homes. If, however, a place of public accommodation, such as a doctor's office or day care center, is located in a private residence, those portions of the residence used for that purpose are subject to the ADA's requirements.

Q. Does the ADA cover air transportation?

A. Discrimination by air carriers in areas other than employment is not covered by the ADA but rather by the Air Carrier Access Act (49 U.S.C. 1374(c)).

Q. What are the ADA's requirements for public transit buses?

A. The Department of Transportation has issued regulations mandating accessible public transit vehicles and facilities. The regulations include requirements that all new fixed-route, public transit buses be accessible and that supplementary paratransit services be provided for those individuals with disabilities who cannot use fixed-route bus service. For information on how to contact the Department of Transportation, see page 170.

Q. How will the ADA make telecommunications accessible?

A. The ADA requires the establishment of telephone relay services for individuals who use telecommunications devices for deaf persons (TDDs) or similar devices. The Federal Communications Commission has issued regulations specifying standards for the operation of these services.

Q. Are businesses entitled to any tax benefit to help pay for the cost of compliance?

A. As amended in 1990, the Internal Revenue Code allows a deduction of up to $15,000 per year for expenses associated with the removal of qualified architectural and transportation barriers. The

1990 amendment also permits eligible small businesses to receive a tax credit for certain costs of compliance with the ADA. An eligible small business is one whose gross receipts do not exceed $1,000,000 or whose workforce does not consist of more than 30 full-time workers. Qualifying businesses may claim a credit of up to 50 percent of eligible access expenditures that exceed $250 but do not exceed $10,250. Examples of eligible access expenditures include the necessary and reasonable costs of removing architectural, physical, communications, and transportation barriers; providing readers, interpreters, and other auxiliary aids; and acquiring or modifying equipment or devices.

Telephone Numbers for ADA Information

This list contains the telephone numbers of Federal agencies that are responsible for providing information to the public about the Americans with Disabilities Act and organizations that have been funded by the Federal government to provide information through staffed information centers. The agencies and organizations listed are sources for obtaining information about the law's requirements and informal guidance in understanding and complying with the ADA.

ADA Information Line
U.S. Department of Justice
For ADA documents and questions
　　800-514-0301 (voice)
　　800-514-0383 (TDD)

Equal Employment Opportunity Commission
For ADA documents
　　800-669-3362 (voice)
　　800-800-3302 (TDD)
For ADA questions
　　800-669-4000 (voice)
　　800-669-6820 (TDD)

U.S. Department of Transportation
ADA documents and information
　　202-366-1656 (voice)
　　202-366-4567 (TDD)
ADA legal questions
　　202-366-1936 (voice)
　　TDD: use relay service

Federal Communications Commission
　　202-418-0190 (voice)
　　202-418-2555 (TDD)

Architectural and Transportation Barriers Compliance Board
　　800-872-2253 (voice)
　　800-993-2822 (TDD)

Job Accommodation Network
　　800-526-7234 (voice)
　　800-526-7234 (TDD)

President's Committee on Employment of People with Disabilities
　　202-376-6200 (voice)
　　202-376-6205 (TDD)

U.S. Department of Education
Regional Disability and Business Technical Assistance Centers
Call automatically connects to your regional center
　　800-949-4232 (voice)
　　800-949-4232 (TDD)

Addresses for ADA Information
U.S. Department of Justice
Civil Rights Division
Disability Rights Section
P.O. Box 66738
Washington, DC 20035-6738

U.S. Equal Employment Opportunity Commission
1801 L Street, NW
Washington, DC 20507

U.S. Department of Transportation
Federal Transit Administration
400 Seventh Street, SW
Washington, DC 20590

Architectural and Transportation Barriers Compliance Board
1331 F Street, NW Suite 1000
Washington, DC 20004-1111

Federal Communications Commission
1919 M Street, NW
Washington, DC 20554

Sample Business Plan

Courtesy of Beth Anderson

MOUNTAIN VIEW REHAB CLINIC
January 2000

Jane Doe
2222 First Street
Anywhere, USA
(715) 999-9999

Table of Contents

MOUNTAIN VIEW REHAB CLINIC

1.1. Mission Statement

MVRC has formulated a mission statement that is reiterated in all our literature to our customers and our employees as well. Our mission statement is as follows: To provide comprehensive, holistic occupational therapy services of direct care (evaluation and treatment), consultation, teaching, and education in a specialized practice.

1.2. Plan Purpose

The purpose of this business plan for MVRC is to acquire financing from a lending institution or a private investor. The total amount needed to start a business of this caliber initially will be $20,000. Jane Doe is investing $5,000 into the business. This investment is for the initial cost of starting a business such as legal fees for forming the corporation plus beginning the process of setting up an office such as rent, supplies, office equipment. Therefore, the company is looking to finance another $15,000 to be used for marketing, technology, and equipment/supplies expenses. Start-up expenses are summarized in section 6.1.

2.0 Company Summary

MVRC has been established as a C-Corporation. The owner is Jane Doe as president. The company was formed on January 15, 2000. The clinic is located in downtown Anywhere in a professional office building. There is free parking and it is conveniently located near a post office, grocery store, and gas station. The office is 2,000 square feet with a reception area, one staff office, and 3 treatment rooms. The office will have state-of-the-art technology such as billing software, electronic billing, computers, fax, voice mail, cell phone, and pager.

3.0   Service Description

The main service provided by MVRC will be occupational therapy (OT). Many areas stem from this therapy: pediatrics or school therapy, hand therapy, industrial services, and wellness programs for companies or individuals. In the industrial industry, many services have been provided by MVRC, including ergonomics assessment, consulting for prevention of cumulative trauma disorders or back injuries.

These services are billed per quarter hour. We are able to bill the following public or private insurance companies for our services: Northwest (Alias) Health Plan; Blue Cross/Blue Shield; Humana; Medicare, and Medicaid. All other area insurances are also accepted. Our office will submit all billing as a service to the customer.

Some future services that MVRC plans to initiate are in-home pediatrics and geriatric OT services. We also plan to launch a new, professional website which will have many functions. It will list services provided by MVRC, educate the general public and medical community on the profession of OT, provide a calendar of related events, and list upcoming continuing education opportunities

4.0   Customer Description

Our customer base has a very large range. Physicians, colleagues, safety directors, teachers, and parents will refer our patients to us. The patients range from all ages, such as school age children to the elderly. Our customers are located in Anywhere and also the outlying seven county areas as well.

Furthermore, we also target companies of all sizes. These services can be worker's compensation claims to safety programs at industrial or manufacturing companies. We would be targeting employees, employers, or more specifically, safety directors within a company. Because of this vast variety, MVRC has a large growth potential.

5.0   Marketing

In this industry, companies thrive on referral or word-of-mouth marketing. Many doctors refer their patients for our services. Other forms of marketing that are used are public radio and newspaper advertisements, and television commercials. Letters are also mailed to physicians offering and explaining our services.

6.0   Management Summary

At our company, Jane Doe is the President, her husband, James, is the Vice President. Being a start-up, we will need to hire the following personnel in order to have a smooth running organization:

1. Office manager: who will organize the overall operations of the office such as filing, appointments, receptionist, bookkeeping.

2. Transcriptionist: who will transcribe all patients' information from the office visit and organize into their file.

As the company grows, we hoped to hire another part-time occupational therapist and an occupational therapy assistant who will divide their duties by outpatient, home visits, and school services.

6.1   Management Team

Jane Doe received her OT certificate from Anonymous University in 1979. Since then, Jane Doe has been in the OT profession for over 20 years. She has also gained experience as a manager of an office, which has helped in the employee relations side of the business. She has worked in a local hospital for 10 years managing the OT team. During this time she received her master's degree in business administration, which has gained her more education and left her as an expert in this field. Her well-rounded knowledge, her education, and work experience has moved her into opening her own clinic.

7.0   Financial Plan

The biggest expense of operating a service company such as this is the high overhead such as equipment, supplies, personnel, rent, etc. This needs to be counterbalanced by a substantial initial investment. Also, a good cash flow is very important in running the company profitably. This is summarized in the next section on start-up costs.

7.1   Start-up Summary

As the table on the following page shows, there are many expenses that are necessary in order to start a business in the OT field. As seen in the table, total start-up expenses are $5,900. However, the biggest initial layout of cash will be for equipment and office furniture of $7,000. This is very important in order to fit the needs of all our customers in the OT industry. Also, there is a cash requirement of $5,000 to leave a good cushion in order to have a strong cash flow at the outset. Therefore, with $5,000 from Jane Doe as an initial investment into her business plan and a short-term loan from the bank for $15,000, this still leaves a Gain of Start-up of $2,100 for any unexpected or underestimated expenses for the initial start-up.

Start-up Expenses

Brochures	$500
Insurance	$500
Legal	$1,000
Office Supplies/Equipment	$2,000
Rent/Damage Deposit	$1,400
Printed Materials	$500
Total Start-up Expenses	$5,900
Start-up Assets Needed	
Cash Requirements	$5,000
Equipment	$5,000
Office Furniture	$2,000
Total Assets Needed	$12,000
Total Cash Needed for Start-up	$17,650
Investment:	
Jane Doe	$5,000
Short-Term Loans/Bank	$15,000
Total Financing	$20,000
Gains/Loss at Start-up	$2,350

Table of Start-up Expenses

7.2   Projected Profit and Loss (See Figure 3.1)

On the next page, there is the three year forecasted profit and loss statement. As it shows, the first year shows a loss as is generally expected in all start-ups because of the initial outlay of expenses to get the company on its feet. However, as the projections show, it will have a steady increase of sales for the next three years as the expenses and salaries show a steady increase as well. It also shows a positive net income in the second year plus a steady increase in the following years. The one expense that is exorbitant in this type of business is the Bad Debt expense which can be high when you are dealing with the health industry. Some people do not have insurance, insurance carriers dispute claims, and/or out-of-pocket expenses to the consumer can be costly. It is our goal to reduce this amount by 10% each year for the next two years in order to have a more positive outlook on our financial statements.

7.3   Projected Balance Sheet (See Figure 1.7)

Licensing and Regulating Agencies

Alabama	Ann Cosby, Executive Director	AL State Board of OT 64 N. Union St., Ste. 734 Montgomery, AL 36130 333-353-4466 (Fax 334-353-4465) E-Mail:
Alaska	Ruth Bluhm, Licensing Examiner	State of Alaska Dept. of Commerce & Economic Development Division of Occupational Licensing State OT & PT Board P.O. Box 110806 Juneau, AL 99811-0806 907-465-3811 (Fax 907-465-2974)
Arizona	Ed Logan, Executive Director	AZ Board of OT Examiners 1400 W. Washington St., Ste. 240 Phoenix, AZ 85007-2931 602-542-6784 (Fax 602-542-5469) E-Mail: azot@primenet.com
Arkansas	Medical Board Licensing Coordinator	AR State Medical Board 2100 Riverfront Drive, Ste 200 Little Rock, AR 72202-1793 501-296-1802 (Fax 501-296-1805)
California (Trademark Law)		OT Association of CA 4600 N. Gate Blvd., Ste 135 Sacramento, CA 95834 916-567-7000

Colorado (Trademark Law)	Linda Graham or Jennifer Whitford, OT	Association of Colorado 809 N. Cascade Ave., Ste C Colorado Springs, CO 80903 719-635-2190 (Fax 719-635-1017) E-Mail: oac99@hotmail.com
Connecticut	Norma Shea or Richard Ouellet	Dept. of Public Health, OT Licensure 410 Capitol Ave., Mail Stop #12APP P.O. Box 340308 Hartford, CT 06134-0308 860-509-7561 (Fax 860-509-8457)
Delaware	Mary Paske, Administrative Assistant	DE State Board of OT Division of Professional Regulation Cannon Bldg., Ste 203 861 Silver Lake Blvd. Dover, DE 19904 302-739-4522, Ext. 207 (Fax 302-739-2711)
District of Columbia	Graphelia Ramseur	DC Board of OT Dept. of Health Office of Professional Licensing 825 N. Capitol St. N.E., Ste. 2224 Washington, D.C. 20002 202-442-9200 (Fax 202-442-9430)
Florida	Debra Boutwell, PRS-II	FL Dept. of Health Board of OT Practice 2020 Capitol Circle S.E. BIN #C05 Tallahassee, FL 32399-3255 850-288-0595 (Fax 850-414-6860) E-Mail: DEB-BOUTSELL@doh.state.fl.us
Georgia	Sandra Marshall	GA Board of OT, Examining Board Division 116 Pryor St., S.W. Atlanta, GA 30303 404-656-3921 (Fax 404-651-9532 or 404-657-2002
Idaho	Nancy Kerr, Executive Director	ID State Board of Medicine P.O. Box 83720, 1755 Westgate Dr., Ste. 140 Boise, ID 83704 208-327-7000 (Fax 208-327-7005
Illinois	Jennifer Witts Allen	Dept. of Professional Regulation, 320 W. Washington St., 3rd Floor Springfield, IL 62786 217-782-8556 (Fax 217-782-7645)
Indiana	Maryann Seyfried, Director of Operations, Kimberly Tarnacki, Deputy Director of Health Prof Bureau	Health Prof Bureau, 402 W. Washington St., 041 Indianapolis, IN 46204 317-232-2960 (Fax 317-233-4236)

Iowa	Judy Manning, Board Administrator	Prof Licensure Office PT & OT Board Examiners Lukas State Office Bldg., Des Moines, IA 50319-0075 – 515-281-7074
Kansas	Rhonda Bohannon, Office Assistant	Kansas State Board of Healing Arts, 235 S. Topeka, Topeka, KA 66603-3068 – 785-296-7413 (Fax 785-296-0852)
Kentucky	Glenda Gordon, Board Administrator	Kentucky OT Board, P.O. Box 1360, Frankfort, KY 40606 – 0456 502-564-2296 (Fax 502-564-4818)
Louisiana	Carol Duchmann	LA State Board of Medical Examiners, 630 Camp St., P.O. Box 30250, New Orleans, LA 70190-0250 504-524-6763 (Fax 504-568-8893)
Maine	Diane Staples, Board Clerk	Dept. of Prof & Financial Regulation, Board of OT Practice, State House Station #35, Augusta, ME 04333 207-624-8626 (Fax 207-582-5415
Maryland	Donna Ashman	MD Board of OT, Spring Grove Hospital Center, Benjamin Rush Bldg. 55 Wade Avenue Baltimore, MD 21228 410-402-8560 (Fax 410-402-8561)
Massachusetts	Kimberly Hamel, Administrative Assist.	Board of Allied Health Professions, Division of Registration 239 Causeway St., Boston, MA 02114 617-627-3071 (Fax 617-727-2197
Michigan	Patricia Lewis	State of MI, Bureau of Health Services P.O. Box 30670 Lansing, MI 48909-7518 517-335-0918 – Applications/Registration 517-373-8102 – Specific OT Questions
Minnesota	Cleone Griep	MN Dept. of Health 121 E. 7th Place, P.O. Box 64975 St. Paul, MN 55164-0975 651-282-5624 (OT/OTA Registration – Mark Meeth)
Mississippi	Stephen Quilter, Health Program Specialist	Professional Licensure MS State Dept. of Health 500 B E. Woodrow Wilson Blvd., Jackson, MS 39216 601-987-4153
Missouri	Desmond Peters, Executive Director	MO Board of OT Box 1335 Jefferson City, MO 65102 573-751-0877

Montana	Helena Lee	Dept. of Commerce MT Board of OT 111 N. Jackson, P.O. Box 200513 Helena, MT 59620-0513 406-444-3091
Nebraska	Brad Rohr	Division of Prof. Licensing Rehab. And Community Services Section Health & Human Services P.O. Box 95007 Lincoln, NE 68509-5007 402-471-0547 or 402-471-4908 (Fax 402-471-0883)
Nevada	Lorraine Pokorski, Executive Secretary	State of NE Board of OT P.O. Box 70220 Reno, NE 89570-0220 775-867-1700 (Fax 775-857-2121)
New Hampshire	Velonique Soucy, Administrative Assist.	NH Board of Allied Health Professions, OT Licensure 2 Industrial Park Drive Concorde, NH 03301 603-271-8389
New Jersey	Laura Anderson, Executive Director	Advisory Council of OT P.O. Box 45037 Newark, NJ 07101 937-504-6570
New Mexico	J.J. Walker	NM Board of OT Practice 2055 S. Pacheco, Ste. 400 P.O. Box 25101 Santa Fe, NM 87505 505-476-7117 (Fax 505-476-7095)
New York	Ronnie Hausheer, Executive Secretary	NY State Board of OT Room 3013 CEC Empire State Plaza Albany, NY 12230 518-473-0221 518-474-3817 – Call for Application
North Carolina	Theresa Kay, Administrative Asst.	NC Board of OT P.O. Box 2280 Raleigh, NC 27602 919-832-1380 (Fax 919-833-1059
North Dakota	Tom Tupa, Adm. Assist. and Ken Tupa, Adm. Assist., Kristin Narum, Executive Secretary	ND State Board of OT Prac. P.O. Box 4005 2900 E. Broadway #5 Bismarck, ND 58502 701-250-0847 phone & fax
Ohio	Carl G. Williams, Executive Director	OH OT, PT and AT Board 77 S. High St., 16th Floor Columbus, OH 43266-0317 614-466-3774 (Fax 614-644-8112

Oklahoma	Kathy Plant, Executive Secretary	Board of Medical Licensure and Supervision P.O. Box 18256 Oklahoma City, OH 73154 405-848-6841 (Fax 405-848-8240
Oregon	Peggy Smith	OT Licensing Board 800 NE Oregon, #21, Ste. 407 Portland, OR 97232 503-731-4048 (Fax 503-731-4207
Pennsylvania	Clara Flinchum, Board Administrator	State Board of OT, Education & Licensure Box 2649 Harrisburg, PA 17105-2649 717-783-1389 (Fax 717-787-7769
Puerto Rico	Beverly Davila, Executive Director	Dept. of Health Office Regulations & Certification of Health Professions Call Box 10200 San Juan, PR 00908 787-725-8121 (Fax 787-725-7903
Rhode Island	Donna Dickerman	Division of Prof. Regulation 3 Capital Hill, Room 104 Providence, RI 02908-5097 401-222-2828, Ext. 106
South Carolina	Brenda M. Owens, Administrator	SC Board of OT 110 Centerview Drive P.O. Box 11329 Columbia, SC 29211-1329 803-896-4683 (Fax 803-896-4719
South Dakota	Mitzi Turley	SD Board of Medical and Osteopathic Examiners 1323 S. Minnesota Ave. Sioux Falls, SD 57105 605-336-1965
Tennessee	Virginia Jenkins Dozier, Lee Phillips	TN Board of OT & PT Examiners 425 Fifth Ave., North Cordell Building, 1st Floor Nashville, TN 37247-1010 615-532-5135 (Fax 615-532-5164
Texas	Cynthia Machado, OT Licensing Sup., Acting Coord. Of OT Programs; Jennifer Jean Jones, Executive Asst., Executive Council of PT and OT Examiners	TX Board of OT Examiners 333 Guadalupe, Ste. 2-510 Austin, TX 78701-3942 512-305-6900 (Fax 512-305-6951
Utah	Karen McCall, Board Secretary	Div. of OT and Prof Licensing 160 E300 South P.O. Box 146741 Salt Lake City, UT 84114-6741 801-530-6632 (Fax 801-530-6511

Vermont	Diane Lafaille, Staff Assist.	Secretary of States Office 109 State Street Montpelier, VT 05609-1106 802-828-2390 (Fax 802-828-2496
Virginia	Cokie Ergens	Virginia Board of Medicine 6606 W. Broad St., 4th Fl. Richmond, VA 23230-1717 804-662-7664
Washington	Carol Neva, Program Manager	Dept. of Health, OT Board P.O. Box 47868 Olympia, WA 98604-7868 360-236-4872 (Fax 360-753-0657
West Virginia	Cathy Whalen	WV Board of OT 119 S. Price St. Kingwood, WV 26537 303-329-0489
Wisconsin	Tammy Buckingham	State of WI Dept. of Regulation & Licensing P.O. Box 8935 Madison, WI 53708-8935 608-266-2112 or 608-266-1396
Wyoming	Vickie L. Spiers, Occupational Licensing Officer	WY Board of OT 116 Logan Ave. Cheyenne, WY 80220 307-432-0488 (Fax 307-432-0492

Sample Informational Column for News Release

LIVING WITH ARTHRITIS

There are many types of arthritis that can affect the quality of our lives. Arthritis pain and stiffness can influence an individual's performance in work, leisure activities and self-care tasks.

If you suffer from arthritis, it doesn't necessarily mean that you need to give up doing things. But you may need to change the way you do some things in order to reduce the amount of "stress" or strain placed on your joints. Overuse and abuse of diseased joints may lead to deformity and loss of function.

If it is important to maintain your present level of activity, ability and independence, there are some basic principles you can follow to prevent unnecessary joint destruction that can occur from daily work and leisure activities.

1. Avoid using muscles or joints in any one position for long periods of time, e.g., holding the telephone, gripping the steering wheel, holding a pen or pencil.
2. Pace activities to include periods of rest.
3. Rest before you get tired.
4. When possible, sit rather than stand or kneel.
5. Use good posture.
6. Learn an appropriate exercise program to move your joints through their normal range of motion. Performing daily exercises will help joint motion and strength.
7. Develop a respect for pain. Do not push joints to or past the point of pain. (The saying, "No pain, no gain" does not apply to arthritis).
8. Never attempt any activity that cannot be stopped immediately if it proves to be beyond your power to complete it, e.g., carrying a bag of groceries, walking up a flight of stairs, transferring a casserole dish from the oven to the table.
9. Organize your work prior to beginning a task so as to eliminate the amount of steps required of a task.
10. Avoid becoming overweight. Excess body weight increases stress placed on joints.
11. Inform your doctor of all medications you use including over the counter drugs and home remedies.
12. Engage in relaxation exercises or guided imagery for pain control.

Some individuals benefit from use of splints to rest their joints or protect them during daily activities. Your physician, chiropractor or therapist can recommend resources for appropriate splints, if necessary.

By incorporating some of these simple techniques in to your daily life, you may be able to reduce some problems associated with arthritis. If you have persistent difficulties engaging in everyday tasks that you were previously able to do or if pain control is unmanageable, you may benefit from a consultation with an Occupational Therapist. We may be able to help you identify ways to perform tasks independently while decreasing the stress placed on your joints.

Elements of Clinical Documentation (Revision)

These elements are provided to assist occupational therapy practitioners to document occupational therapy services. Occupational therapy practitioners determine the appropriate type of documentation and document the services provided within the time frames established by facilities, government agencies, and accreditation organizations. These elements do not address the specific content of documentation which is unique to occupational therapy intervention for particular ages and types of impairments.

The purpose of documentation is to:

1. Provide a chronological record of the consumer's condition which details the complete course of therapeutic intervention.

2. Facilitate communication among professionals who contribute to the consumer's care.

3. Provide an objective basis to determine the appropriateness, effectiveness, and necessity of therapeutic intervention.

4. Reflect the practitioner's reasoning.

Types of Documentation

    I. Evaluation Report

       A. Identification and Background Information

       B. Assessment Results

       C. Intervention or Treatment Plan

   II. Contact, Treatment, or Visit Note

 III. Progress Report

 IV. Re-evaluation Report

   V. Discharge or Discontinuation Report

Source: AOTA, 1995.

Prepared by Linda Kohlman Thomson, OT, OTR, OT(C), FAOTA, Mary Foto, OTR, FAOTA, for the Commission on Practice (Jim Hinojosa, PhD., OTR, FAOTA. Chairperson).

Approved by the Representative Assembly April 1986.

Revised 1994 and sent to the Representative Assembly FYI.

This document replaces the 1986 Guidelines for Occupational Therapy Documentation. (American Journal of Occupational Therapy, 40, 830-832).

Note: If a document is revised, the previous version is superseded and, according to Parliamentary procedure, is automatically rescinded.

I. Evaluation Report

Used to document the initial contact with the consumer, the data collected, the interpretation of the data, and the intervention plan. When an abbreviated evaluation process is used, such as screening, it is documented using only limited content areas applicable to the consumer and situation.

    A. Identification and Background Information (See Table 1)

    B. Assessment Results (see Table 2)

    C. Intervention or Treatment Plan (see Table 3)

Table 1   Identification and Background Information

CONTENT	CLARIFICATION
1. Name, age, sex, date of admission, treatment diagnosis, and date of onset of current diagnosis	Name may be omitted, depending on facility and department policies and procedures.
2. Referral source, services requested, and date of referral to occupational therapy	Who requested occupational therapy services, what specific services were requested, and date services were requested.
3. Medical history and secondary problems or preexisting conditions, prior therapy	Additional problems or conditions that may affect consumer function outcomes.
4. Precautions and contraindications	May be identified by referral source or occupational therapy practitioners.
5. Pertinent history that indicates prior levels of function and support systems	Applicable development of educational, vocational, cultural, and socioeconomic history.
6. Present levels of function in performance areas determined by examination*	Brief description of the consumer's level of performance in activities of daily living, work and productive activities, and play or leisure activities.
7. Performance contexts determined by examination*	Description of those temporal aspects (chronological, developmental, life cycle, health status) and environmental (physical, social, cultural) features that affect the consumer's function in performance areas.
8. Consumer and family expectations	Brief description of expected outcome of occupational therapy intervention.

*Refer to *Uniform Terminology for Occupational Therapy*, Third Edition (AOTA, 1994a), for specific performance areas, performance components, and performance contexts.

II. Contact, Treatment, or Visit Note

Used to document individual occupational therapy session or care coordination. May be very brief, such as in the use of a checklist, flow chart, or short narrative-type notation (see Table 4).

Table 2   Assessment Results

CONTENT	CLARIFICATION
1. Tests and assessments administered and the results	Name and type of assessment or test and the results: may include comparison with previous testing. State if standardized procedure not followed.
2. References to other pertinent reports and information	Any additional sources of data or assessment results used.
3. Summary and analysis of evaluation findings	State the type and severity of impairments identified and the functional limitations caused by the impairments in objective, functional, and measurable terms. Include the functional diagnosis.
4. Projected functional outcome(s)	Prognosis and anticipated level of performance (activities of daily living [ADL], work or productive activities, and play or leisure activities) the consumer will be able to achieve as a result of therapeutic intervention. May include a statement indicating the consumer does not have the potential to improve beyond current status.

III. Progress Report

Used periodically to document care coordination, interventions, progress toward functional goals, and to update goals and intervention or treatment plan (see Table 5).

IV Re-evaluation Report

Used to document sessions in which portions of the evaluation process are repeated or readministered. Usually occurs monthly or quarterly, depending on the setting (see Table 6).

V. Discharge or Discontinuation Report

Used to document a summary of the course of therapy and any recommendations (see Table 7).

Fundamental Elements of Documentation

Each consumer of occupational therapy services must have a case record maintained as a permanent file. The record should be organized, legible, concise, clear, accurate, complete, current, and objective. Correct grammar and spelling should be used.

The following 10 elements should be present:

1. Consumer's full name and case number on each page of documentation.

2. Date stated as month, day, and year for each entry; time of intervention; and length of session.

3. Identification of type of documentation and department name.

Table 3   Intervention or Treatment Plan

CONTENT	CLARIFICATION
1. Long-term functional goals	Functional limitations that must change in order to achieve the projected functional outcome. Degree the functional limitations will be decreased. Rationale for decreasing functional limitations. Functional change to occur by end of intervention. Consumer and/or family agreement with goals.
2. Short-term goals	Directly relate to long-term functional goals. Impairment that must change in order to achieve the projected functional outcome. Degree the impairment will be decreased. Functional ability that will result from a decrease in level of impairment. Change to occur in a brief period of time (e.g., 7, 14, or 30 days). Consumer and/or family agreement with goals.
3. Intervention or treatment procedures	Activities, techniques, and modalities selected to be used and how they relate to goals. May include family training and home programs. Identify assistive/adaptive equipment, orthotics, and/or prosthetics to meet consumer's environmental adaptation needs.
4. Type, amount, frequency, and duration of intervention or treatment	State skill and performance areas to be addressed and estimate the number, duration, and frequency of sessions to accomplish goals.
5. Recommendations	Need for OT services and necessary referrals to other professionals.

Table 4   Contact, Treatment, or Visit Note

CONTENT	CLARIFICATION
1. Attendance and participation	Therapy occurrence or reason for therapy not occurring as scheduled.
2. Activities, techniques, and modalities used	May be indicated by checklist or brief statement.
3. Assistive adaptive equipment, prosthetics, and orthotics if issued or fabricated, and specific instructions for the application and/or use of the item	State the device; note whether it was fabricated, sold, rented, or loaned; and state the effectiveness of the device.
4. Consumer's response to therapy	Level of performance and anything unusual or significant that was a result of occupational therapy intervention.

Table 5   Progress Report

CONTENT	CLARIFICATION
1. Activities, techniques, and modalities used	Brief statement of intervention process.
2. Consumer's response to therapy, and the progress toward short-and long-term goal attainment and comparison with previous functional status	State the consumer's physical and behavioral response to therapy, whether the goals are being achieved, if change has occurred, and how much change has occurred.
3. Goal continuance	Explanation for no or slow progress, reason for not meeting short-term goal(s), or need to continue current goal(s).
4. Goal modification when indicated by the response to therapy or by the establishment of new consumer needs	State new goals and rationale for changes or additions.
5. Change in anticipated time to achieve goals	If, for any reason, the therapy time frame is altered, include the reason for the change and the new anticipated time frame.
6. Assistive/adaptive equipment, prosthetics, and orthotics, if issued or fabricated, and specific instructions for the application and/or use of the item.	State the device; note whether it was fabricated, sold, rented, or loaned; and state the effectiveness of the device.
7. Consumer-related conferences and communication	If occupational therapy practitioners participated in a conference or made a pertinent contact with a family member, agency, or health care professional, state this information with a brief summary of the conference or communication.
8. Home programs	Include a copy of the home program as established with the consumer. Include a statement regarding the consumer's ability to follow the program.
9. Consumer/caretaker instruction	What instruction was provided and in what format (i.e., verbal or written).
10. Plan	Specific procedures, communication, or consultations to be done in the future to address the goals.

4. Practitioner's signature with a minimum of first name of initial, last name, and professional designation.

5. Signature of the recorder directly at the end of the note without space left between the body of the note and the signature.

6. Countersignature by a registered occupational therapist (OTR) on documentation written by students and certified occupational therapy assistants (COTA) when required by law of the facility.

7. Compliance with confidentiality standards.

8. Acceptable terminology as defined by the facility.

Table 6 Re-evaluation Report

CONTENT	CLARIFICATION
1. Tests and assessments readministered and the results	Name and type of test readministered. State if standardized procedure is not followed.
2. Comparative summary and analysis of previous evaluation findings	Results analyzed and compared with previous testing.
3. Reestablishment of projected functional outcome(s)	Anticipated level of performance (ADL, work or productive activities, and play or leisure activities) the consumer will be able to achieve as a result of therapeutic intervention. May include a statement of changes in previously established functional outcome(s) based on revised potential or goals of consumer.
4. Update of intervention or treatment plan	Revised or continued long-term functional goals; short-term goals; treatment procedures; and type, amount, and frequency of therapy.

Table 7 Discharge or Discontinuation Report

CONTENT	CLARIFICATION
1. Therapy process	Summary of interventions used, consumer's responses, and number of sessions.
2. Goal attainment	Degree to which short- and long-term functional goals were achieved.
3. Functional outcome	Comparison of functional status prior to therapy and at discharge.
4. Home programs	Include the actual written home program that is to be followed after discharge.
5. Follow-up plans	State the schedule and specific plans.
6. Recommendations	State any recommendations pertaining to the consumer's future needs.
7. Referral(s) to other health care providers and community agencies	Indicate referral(s) or recommendations for referral(s) when additional or new services are needed.

9. Facility-approved abbreviations.

10. Errors corrected by drawing a single line through an error, and the correction initialed (liquid correction fluid and erasures are not acceptable), or facility requirements followed.

References

American Occupational Therapy Association. (1994a). Uniform terminology for occupational therapy – Third edition. *American Journal of Occupational Therapy, 48,* 1047-1054.

American Occupational Therapy Association. (1994b). Uniform terminology – Third edition: Application to practice. *American Journal of Occupational Therapy, 48,* 1055-1059.

Bibliography

Allen, C. K., Earhart, C .A., & Blue, T. (1992). *Occupational therapy treatment goals for the physically and cognitively disabled.* Bethesda, MD: American Occupational Therapy Association.

Allen, C., Foto, M., Moon-Sperling, T. & Wilson, D. (Eds.). (December 1989). A medical review approach to medicare outpatient documentation. *American Journal of Occupational Therapy, 43,* 793-800.

American Occupational Therapy Association. (1989). Reports that work. *AOTA self study series: Assessing function* (Chapter 9). Bethesda, MD: Author.

American Occupational Therapy Association. (1992). *Effective documentation for occupational therapy.* Bethesda, MD: Author.

American Occupational Therapy Association. (1994). Standards of practice for occupational therapy. *American Journal of Occupational Therapy, 48,* 1039-1043.

Hopkins, H. L., & Smith, H. D. (1993). *Willard and Spackman's occupational therapy* (8th ed.). Philadelphia: Lippincott.

Stewart, D. L., & Abeln, S. H. (Eds.). (1993). *Documenting functional outcomes in physical therapy.* St. Louis: Mosby.

Uniform Terminology for Occupational Therapy— Third Edition

This is an official document of the American Occupational Therapy Association (AOTA). This document is intended to provide a generic outline of the domain of concern of occupational therapy and is designed to create common terminology for the profession and to capture the essence of occupational therapy succinctly for others.

It is recognized that the phenomena that constitute the profession's domain of concern can be categorized, and labeled, in a number of different ways. This document is not meant to limit those in the field, formulating theories or frames of reference, who may wish to combine or refine particular constructs. It is also not meant to limit those who would like to conceptualize the profession's domain of concern in a different manner.

Introduction

The first edition of Uniform Terminology was approved and published in 1979 (AOTA, 1979). In 1989, *Uniform Terminology for Occupational Therapy—Second Edition* (AOTA, 1989) was approved and published. The second document presented an organized structure for understanding the areas of practice for the profession of occupational therapy. The document outlined two domains. Performance areas (activities of daily living [ADL], work and productive activities, and play or leisure) include activities that the occupational therapy practitioner emphasizes when determining functional abilities (occupational therapy practitioner refers to both registered occupational therapists and certified occupational therapy assistants). Performance

Source: AOTA, 1994.

Prepared by The Terminology Task Force: Winifred Dunn, PhD., OTR, FAOTA, Chairperson; Mary Foto, OTR, FAOTA; Jim Hinojosa, PhD., OTR, FAOTA; Barbara Schell, PhD., OTR/L, FAOTA; Linda Kohlman Thomson, MOT, OTR, FAOTA; Sarah D. Hertfelder, Med., MOT, OTR1 — Staff Liaison, for the Commission on Practice (Jim Hinojosa, PhD., OTR, FAOTA, Chairperson).

Adopted by the Representative Assembly July 1994.

This document replaces the following documents, all of which were rescinded by the 1994 Representative Assembly; Occupational Therapy Product Output Reporting System *(1979),* Uniform Terminology for Reporting Occupational Therapy Services — First Edition *(1979), "Uniform Occupational Therapy Evaluation Checklist" (1981, American Journal of Occupational Therapy, 35, 817-818), and "Uniform Terminology for Occupational Therapy — Second Edition" (1989, American Journal of Occupational Therapy, 43, 808-815).*

components (sensorimotor, cognitive, psychosocial, and psychological aspects) are the elements of performance that occupational therapists assess and, when needed, in which they intervene for improved performance.

This third edition has been further expanded to reflect current practice and to incorporate contextual aspects of performance. Performance areas, performance components, and performance contexts are the parameters of occupational therapy's domain of concern. Performance areas are broad categories of human activity that are typically part of daily life. They are activities of daily living, work and productive activities, and play or leisure activities. Performance components are fundamental human abilities that—to varying degrees and in differing combinations—are required for successful engagement in performance areas. These components are sensorimotor, cognitive, psychosocial, and psychological. Performance contexts are situations or factors that influence an individual's engagement in desired and/or required performance areas. Performance contexts consist of temporal aspects (chronological age, developmental age, place in the life cycle, and health status) and environmental aspects (physical, social, and cultural considerations). There is an interactive relationship among performance areas, performance components, and performance contexts. Function in performance areas is the ultimate concern of occupational therapy, with performance components considered as they relate to participation in performance areas. Performance areas and performance components are always viewed within performance contexts. Performance contexts are taken into consideration when determining function and dysfunction relative to performance areas and performance components, and in planning intervention. For example, the occupational therapist does not evaluate strength (a performance component) in isolation. Strength is considered as it affects necessary or desired tasks (performance areas). If the individual is interested in homemaking, the occupational therapy practitioner would consider the interaction of strength with homemaking tasks. Strengthening could be addressed through kitchen activities, such as cooking and putting groceries away. In some cases, the practitioner would employ an adaptive approach and recommend that the family switch from heavy stoneware to lighter-weight dishes, or use lighter-weight pots on the stove to enable the individual to make dinner

safely without becoming fatigued or compromising safety.

Occupational therapy assessment involves examining performance areas, performance components, and performance contexts. Intervention may be directed toward elements of performance areas (e.g., dressing, vocational exploration), performance components (e.g., endurance, problem solving), or the environmental aspects of performance contexts. In the latter case, the physical and/or social environment may be altered or augmented to improve and/or maintain function. After identifying the performance areas the individual wishes or needs to address, the occupational therapist assesses the features of the environments in which the tasks will be performed. If an individual's job requires cooking in a restaurant as opposed to leisure cooking at home, the occupational therapy practitioner faces several challenges to enable the individual's success in different environments. Therefore, the third critical aspect of performance is the performance context, the features of the environment that affect the person's ability to engage in functional activities.

This document categorizes specific activities in each of the performance areas (ADL, work and productive activities, play or leisure). This categorization is based on what is considered "typical," and is not meant to imply that a particular individual characterizes personal activities in the same manner as someone else. Occupational therapy practitioners embrace individual differences, and so would document the unique pattern of the individual being served, rather than forcing the "typical" pattern on him or her and family. For example, because of experience or culture, a particular individual might think of home management as an ADL task rather than "work and productive activities" (current listing). Socialization might be considered part of a play or leisure activity instead of its current listing as part of "activities of daily living," because of life experience or cultural heritage.

Examples of Use in Practice

Uniform Terminology—Third Edition defines occupational therapy's domain of concern, which includes performance areas, performance components, and performance contexts. While this document may be used by occupational therapy practitioners in a number of different areas (e.g., practice, documentation, charge systems, education, program development, marketing, research, disability classifications, and regulations), it focuses on the use of uniform terminology in practice. This document is not intended to define specific occupational therapy programs or specific occupational therapy interventions. Examples of how performance areas, performance components, and performance contexts translate into practice are provided below.

- An individual who is injured on the job may have the potential to return to work and productive activities, which is a performance area. In order to achieve the outcome of returning to work and productive activities, the individual may need to address specific performance components, such as strength, endurance, soft tissue integrity, time management, and the physical features of performance contexts, like structures and objects in his or her environment. The occupational therapy practitioner, in collaboration with the individual and other members of the vocational team, uses planned interventions to achieve the desired outcome. These interventions may include activities such as an exercise program, body mechanics instruction, and job site modifications, all of which may be provided in a work-hardening program.

- An elderly individual recovering from a cerebro-vascular accident may wish to live in a community setting, which combines the performance areas of ADL with work and productive activities. In order to achieve the outcome of community living, the individual may need to address specific performance components, such as muscle tone, gross motor coordination, postural control, and self management. It is also necessary to consider the sociocultural and physical features of performance contexts, such as support available from other persons, and adaptations of structures and objects within the environment. The occupational therapy practitioner, in cooperation with the team, utilizes planned interventions to achieve the desired outcome. Interventions may include neuromuscular facilitation, practice of object manipulation,

and instruction in the use of adaptive equipment and home safety equipment. The practitioner and individual also pursue the selection and training of a personal assistant to ensure the completion of ADL tasks. These interventions may be provided in a comprehensive inpatient rehabilitation unit.

- A child with learning disabilities is required to perform educational activities within a public school setting. Engaging in educational activities is considered the performance area of work and productive activities for this child. To achieve the educational outcome of efficient and effective completion of written classroom work, the child may need to address specific performance components. These include sensory processing, perceptual skills, postural control, motor skills, and the physical features of performance contexts, such as objects (e.g., desk, chair) in the environment. In cooperation with the team, occupational therapy interventions may include activities like adapting the student's seating in the classroom to improve postural control and stability, and practicing motor control and coordination. This program could be developed by an occupational therapist and supported by school district personnel.

- The parents of an infant with cerebral palsy may ask to facilitate the child's involvement in the performance areas of activities of daily living and play. Subsequent to assessment, the therapist identifies specific performance components, such as sensory awareness and neuromuscular control. The practitioner also addresses the physical and cultural features of performance contexts. In collaboration with the parents, occupational therapy interventions may include activities such as seating and positioning for play, neuromuscular facilitation techniques to enable eating, facilitating parent skills in caring for and playing with their infant, and modifying the play space for accessibility. These interventions may be provided in a home-based occupational therapy program.

- An adult with schizophrenia may need and want to live independently in the community, which represents the performance areas of activities of daily living, work and productive activities, and leisure activities. The specific performance categories may be medication routine, functional mobility, home management, vocational exploration, play or leisure performance, and social interaction. In order to achieve the outcome of living independently, the individual may need to address specific performance components, such as topographical orientation; memory; categorization; problem solving; interests; social conduct; time management; and sociocultural features of performance contexts, such as social factors (e.g., influence of family and friends) and roles. The occupational therapy practitioner, in cooperation with the team, utilizes planned interventions to achieve the desired outcome. Interventions may include activities such as training in the use of public transportation, instruction in budgeting skills, selection and participation in social activities, instruction in social conduct, and participation in community reintegration activities. These interventions may be provided in a community-based mental health program.

- An individual with a history of substance abuse may need to reestablish family roles and responsibilities, which represent the performance areas of activities of daily living, work and productive activities, and leisure activities. In order to achieve the outcome of family participation, the individual may need to address the performance components of roles; values; social conduct; self-expression; coping skills; self-control; and the sociocultural features of performance contexts, such as custom, behavior, rules, and rituals. The occupational therapy practitioner, in cooperation with the team, utilizes planned interventions to achieve the desired outcomes. Interventions may include roles and values exercises, instruction in stress management techniques, identification of family roles and activities, and support to develop family leisure routines. These interventions may be provided in an inpatient acute care unit.

Person-Activity-Environment Fit

Person-activity-environment fit refers to the match among the skills and abilities of the individual; the demands of the activity; and the characteristics of the physical, social, and cultural environments. It is the interaction among the performance areas, performance components, and performance contexts that is important and determines the success of the performance. When occupational therapy practitioners provide services, they attend to all of these aspects of performance and the interaction among them. They also attend to each individual's unique personal history. The personal history includes one's skills and abilities (performance components), the past performance of specific life tasks (performance areas), and experience within particular environments (performance contexts). In addition to personal history, anticipated life tasks and role demands influence performance.

When considering the person-activity-environment fit, variables such as novelty, importance, motivation, activity tolerance, and quality are salient. Situations range from those that are completely familiar to those that are novel and have never been experienced. Both the novelty and familiarity within a situation contribute to the overall task performance. In each situation, there is an optimal level of novelty that engages the individual sufficiently and provides enough information to perform the task. When too little novelty is present, the individual may miss cues and opportunities to perform. When too much novelty is present, the individual may become confused and distracted, inhibiting effective task performance.

Humans determine that some stimuli and situations are more meaningful than others. Individuals perform tasks they deem important. It is critical to identify what the individual wants or needs to do when planning interventions.

The level of motivation an individual demonstrates to perform a particular task is determined by both internal and external factors. An individual's biobehavioral state (e.g., amount of rest, arousal, tension) contributes to the potential to be responsive. The features of the social and physical environments (e.g., persons in the room, noise level) provide information that is either adequate or inadequate to produce a motivated state.

Activity tolerance is the individual's ability to sustain a purposeful activity over time.

Individuals must not only select, initiate, and terminate activities, but they must also attend to a task for the needed length of time to complete the task and accomplish their goals.

The quality of performance is measured by standards generated by both the individual and others in the social and cultural environments in which the performance occurs. Quality is a continuum of expectations set within particular activities and contexts (see Figure 1).

Uniform Terminology for Occupational Therapy—Third Edition

Occupational therapy is the use of purposeful activity interventions to promote health and achieve functional outcomes. Achieving functional outcomes means to develop, improve, or restore the highest possible level of independence of any individual who is limited by a physical injury or illness, a dysfunctional condition, a cognitive impairment, a psychosocial dysfunction, a mental illness, a developmental or learning disability, or an adverse environmental condition. Assessment means the use of skilled observation or evaluation by the administration and interpretation of standardized or nonstandardized tests and measurements to identify areas for occupational therapy services.

Occupational therapy services include, but are not limited to

1. the assessment, treatment, and education of or consultation with the individual, family, or other persons; or

2. interventions directed toward developing, improving, or restoring daily living skills, work readiness or work performance, play skills or leisure capacities, or enhancing educational performance skills; or

3. providing for the development, improvement, or restoration of sensorimotor, oral-motor, perceptual or neuromuscular functioning; or emotional, motivational, cognitive, or psychosocial components of performance.

These services may require assessment of the need for and use of interventions such as the design, development, adaptation, application, or training in the use of assistive technology devices, the design, fabrication, or application of rehabilitative technology such as selected orthotic devices; training in the use of assistive technology, orthotic or prosthetic devices; the application of physical agent modalities as an adjunct to or in preparation for purposeful activity, the use of ergonomic principles, the adaptation of environments and processes to enhance functional performance; or the promotion of health and wellness (AOTA, 1993, p. 1117).

I. Performance Areas

Throughout this document, activities have been described as if individuals performed the tasks themselves. Occupational therapy also recognizes that individuals arrange for tasks to be done through others. The profession views independence as the ability to self-determine activity performance, regardless of who actually performs the activity.

A. *Activities of Daily Living*—Self-maintenance tasks.

1. *Grooming*—Obtaining and using supplies; removing body hair (use of razors, tweezers, lotions, etc.); applying and removing cosmetics; washing, drying, combing, styling, and brushing hair; caring for nails (hands and feet), caring for skin, ears, and eyes; and applying deodorant.

2. *Oral Hygiene*—Obtaining and using supplies; cleansing mouth; brushing and flossing teeth; or removing, cleaning, and reinserting dental orthotics and prosthetics.

3. *Bathing/Showering*—Obtaining and using supplies; soaping, rinsing, and drying body parts; maintaining bathing position; and transferring to and from bathing positions.

4. *Toilet Hygiene*—Obtaining and using supplies; clothing management; maintaining toileting position; transferring to and from toileting position; cleaning body; and caring for menstrual and continence needs (including catheters, colostomies, and suppository management).

5. *Personal Device Care*—Cleaning and maintaining personal care items, such as hearing aids, contact lenses, glasses, orthotics, prosthetics, adaptive equipment, and contraceptive and sexual devices.

I. Performance Areas
- A. Activities of Daily Living
    1. Grooming
    2. Oral Hygiene
    3. Bathing/Showering
    4. Toilet Hygiene
    5. Personal Device Care
    6. Dressing
    7. Feeding and Eating
    8. Medication Routine
    9. Health Maintenance
    10. Socialization
    11. Functional Communication
    12. Functional Mobility
    13. Community Mobility
    14. Emergency Response
    15. Sexual Expression
- B. Work and Productive Activities
    1. Home Management
        a. Clothing Care
        b. Cleaning
        c. Meal Preparation/Cleanup
        d. Shopping
        e. Money Management
        f. Household Maintenance
        g. Safety Procedures
    2. Care of Others
    3. Educational Activities
    4. Vocational Activities
        a. Vocational Exploration
        b. Job Acquisition
        c. Work or Job Performance
        d. Retirement Planning
        e. Volunteer Participation
- C. Play or Leisure Activities
    1. Play or Leisure Exploration
    2. Play or Leisure Performance

II. Performance Components
- A. Sensorimotor Component
    1. Sensory
        a. Sensory Awareness
        b. Sensory Processing
            (1) Tactile
            (2) Proprioceptive
            (3) Vestibular
            (4) Visual
            (5) Auditory
            (6) Gustatory
            (7) Olfactory
        c. Perceptual Processing
            (1) Stereognosis
            (2) Kinesthesia
            (3) Pain Response
            (4) Body Scheme
            (5) Right-left Discrimination
            (6) Form Constancy
            (7) Position in Space
            (8) Visual-Closure
            (9) Figure Ground
            (10) Depth Perception
            (11) Spatial Relations
            (12) Topographical Orientation
    2. Neuromusculoskeletal
        a. Reflex
        b. Range of Motion
        c. Muscle Tone
        d. Strength
        e. Endurance
        f. Postural Control
        g. Postural Alignment
        h. Soft Tissue Integrity
    3. Motor
        a. Gross Coordination
        b. Crossing the Midline
        c. Laterally
        d. Bilateral Integration
        e. Motor Control
        f. Praxis
        g. Fine Coordination/Dexterity
        h. Visual-Motor Integration
        i. Oral-Motor Control
- B. Cognitive Integration and Cognitive Components
    1. Level of Arousal
    2. Orientation
    3. Recognition
    4. Attention Span

Figure 1. Uniform Terminology for Occupational Therapy—Third Edition outline (*continues*)

5. Initiation of Activity
6. Termination of Activity
7. Memory
8. Sequencing
9. Categorization
10. Concept Formation
11. Spatial Operations
12. Problem Solving
13. Learning
14. Generalization

C. Psychosocial Skills and Psychological
Components
  1. Psychological
    a. Values
    b. Interests
    c. Self-Concept
  2. Social
    a. Role Performance
    b. Social Conduct
    c. Interpersonal Skills
    d. Self-Expression
  3. Self-Management
    a. Coping Skills
    b. Time Management
    c. Self-Control

III. Performance Contexts
A. Temporal Aspects
  1. Chronological
  2. Developmental
  3. Life Cycle
  4. Disability Status

B. Environment
  1. Physical
  2. Social
  3. Cultural

Figure 1. Uniform Terminology for Occupational Therapy—Third Edition outline (*continued*)

6. *Dressing*—Selecting clothing and accessories appropriate to time of day, weather, and occasion; obtaining clothing from storage area; dressing and undressing in a sequential fashion; fastening and adjusting clothing and shoes; and applying and removing personal devices, prostheses, or orthoses.

7. *Feeding and Eating*—Setting up food; selecting and using appropriate utensils and tableware; bringing food or drink to mouth; cleaning face, hands, and clothing; sucking, masticating, coughing, and swallowing; and management of alternative methods of nourishment.

8. *Medication Routine*—Obtaining medication, opening and closing containers, following prescribed schedules, taking correct quantities, reporting problems and adverse effects, and administering correct quantities by using prescribed methods.

9. *Health Maintenance*—Developing and maintaining routines for illness prevention and wellness promotion, such as physical fitness, nutrition, and decreasing health risk behaviors.

10. *Socialization*—Accessing opportunities and interacting with other people in appropriate contextual and cultural ways to meet emotional and physical needs.

11. *Functional Communication*—Using equipment or systems to send and receive information, such as writing equipment, telephones, typewriters, computers, communication boards, call lights, emergency systems, Braille writers, telecommunication devices for the deaf, and augmentative communication systems.

12. *Functional Mobility*—Moving from one position or place to another, such as in-bed mobility, wheelchair mobility, transfers (wheelchair, bed, car, tub, toilet, tub/shower, chair, floor). Performing functional ambulation and transporting objects.

13. *Community Mobility*—Moving self in the community and using public or private

transportation, such as driving, or accessing buses, taxi cabs, or other public transportation systems.

14. *Emergency Response*—Recognizing sudden, unexpected hazardous situations, and initiating action to reduce the threat to health and safety.

15. *Sexual Expression*—Engaging in desired sexual and intimate activities.

B. *Work and Productive Activities*—Purposeful activities for self-development, social contribution, and livelihood.

1. *Home Management*—Obtaining and maintaining personal and household possessions and environment.

    a. *Clothing care*—Obtaining and using supplies; sorting, laundering (hand, machine, and dry clean); folding; ironing; storing; and mending.

    b. *Cleaning*—Obtaining and using supplies; picking up; putting away; vacuuming; sweeping and mopping floors; dusting; polishing; scrubbing; washing windows; cleaning mirrors; making beds; and removing trash and recyclables.

    c. *Meal Preparation and Cleanup*—Planning nutritious meals; preparing and serving food; opening and closing containers, cabinets and drawers; using kitchen utensils and appliances; cleaning up and storing food safely.

    d. *Shopping*—Preparing shopping lists (grocery and other); selecting and purchasing items; selecting method of payment; and completing money transactions.

    e. *Money Management*—Budgeting, paying bills, and using bank systems.

    f. *Household Maintenance*—Maintaining home, yard, garden, appliances, vehicles, and household items.

    g. *Safety Procedures*—Knowing and performing preventive and emergency procedures to maintain a safe environment and to prevent injuries.

2. *Care of Others*—Providing for children, spouse, parents, pets, or others, such as giving physical care, nurturing, communicating, and using age-appropriate activities.

3. *Educational Activities*—Participating in a learning environment through school, community, or work-sponsored activities, such as exploring educational interests, attending to instruction, managing assignments, and contributing to group experiences.

4. *Vocational Activities*—Participating in work-related activities.

    a. *Vocational Exploration*—Determining attitudes; developing interests and skills, and selecting appropriate vocational pursuits.

    b. *Job Acquisition*—Identifying and selecting work opportunities, and completing application and interview processes.

    c. *Work or Job Performance*—Performing job tasks in a timely and effective manner; incorporating necessary work behaviors.

    d. *Retirement Planning*—Determining aptitudes; developing interests and skills, and selecting appropriate avocational pursuits.

    e. *Volunteer Participation*—Performing unpaid activities for the benefit of selected individuals, groups, or causes.

C. *Play or Leisure Activities*—Intrinsically motivating activities for amusement, relaxation, spontaneous enjoyment, or self-expression.

1. *Play or Leisure Exploration*—Identifying interests, skills, opportunities, and appropriate play or leisure activities.

2. *Play or Leisure Performance*—Planning and participating in play or leisure activities. Maintaining a balance of play or leisure activities with work and productive activities, and activities of daily living. Obtaining, utilizing, and maintaining equipment and supplies.

II. Performance Components

A. *Sensorimotor Component*—The ability to receive input, process information, and produce output.

1. *Sensory*

    a. *Sensory Awareness*—Receiving and differentiating sensory stimuli.

b. *Sensory Processing*—Interpreting sensory stimuli:
1) *Tactile*—Interpreting light touch, pressure, temperature, pain, and vibration through skin contact/receptors.
2) *Proprioceptive*—Interpreting stimuli originating in muscles, joints, and other internal tissues that give information about the position of one body part in relation to another.
3) *Vestibular*—Interpreting stimuli from the inner ear receptors regarding head position and movement.
4) *Visual*—Interpreting stimuli through the eyes, including peripheral vision and acuity, and awareness of color and pattern.
5) *Auditory*—Interpreting and localizing sounds, and discriminating background sounds.
6) *Gustatory*—Interpreting tastes.
7) *Olfactory*—Interpreting odors.

c. *Perceptual Processing*—Organizing sensory input into meaningful patterns.
1) *Stereognosis*—Identifying objects through proprioception, cognition, and the sense of touch.
2) *Kinesthesia*—Identifying objects through proprioception, cognition, and the sense of touch.
3) *Pain Response*—Interpreting noxious stimuli.
4) *Body Scheme*—Acquiring an internal awareness of the body and the relationship of body parts to each other.
5) *Right-Left Discrimination*—Differentiating one side from the other.
6) *Form Constancy*—Recognizing forms and objects as the same in various environments, positions, and sizes.
7) *Position in Space*—Determining the spatial relationship of figures and objects to self or other forms and objects.
8) *Visual-Closure*—Identifying forms or objects from incomplete presentations.
9) *Figure Ground*—Differentiating between foreground and background forms and objects.
10) *Depth Perception*—Determining the relative distance between objects, figures, or landmarks and the observer, and changes in planes of surfaces.
11) *Spatial Relations*—Determining the position of objects relative to each other.
12) *Topographical Orientation*—Determining the location of objects and settings and the route to the location.

2. *Neuromusculoskeletal*
a. *Reflex*—Eliciting an involuntary muscle response by sensory input.
b. *Range of Motion*—Moving body parts through an arc.
c. *Muscle Tone*—Demonstrating a degree of tension or resistance in a muscle at rest and in response to stretch.
d. *Strength*—Demonstrating a degree of muscle power when movement is resisted, as with objects or gravity.
e. *Endurance*—Sustaining cardiac, pulmonary, and musculoskeletal exertion over time.
f. *Postural Control*—Using righting and equilibrium adjustments to maintain balance during functional movements.
g. *Postural Alignment*—Maintaining biomechanical integrity among body parts.
h. *Soft Tissue Integrity*—Maintaining anatomical and physiological condition of interstitial tissue and skin.

3. *Motor*
a. *Gross Coordination*—Using large muscle groups for controlled, goal-directed movements.
b. *Crossing the Midline*—Moving limbs and eyes across the midsagittal plane of the body.
c. *Laterality*—Using a preferred unilateral body part for activities requiring a high level of skill.
d. *Bilateral Integration*—Coordinating both body sides during activity.

e. *Motor Control*—Using the body in functional and versatile movement patterns.

f. *Praxis*—Conceiving and planning a new motor act in response to an environmental demand.

g. *Fine Coordination/Dexterity*—Using small muscle groups for controlled movements, particularly in object manipulation.

h. *Visual-Motor Integration*—Coordinating the interaction of information from the eyes with body movement during activity.

i. *Oral-Motor Control*—Coordinating oropharyngeal musculature for controlled movements.

B. *Cognitive Integration and Cognitive Components*—The ability to use higher brain functions.

1. *Level of Arousal*—Demonstrating alertness and responsiveness to environmental stimuli.

2. *Orientation*—Identifying person, place, time, and situation.

3. *Recognition*—Identifying familiar faces, objects, and other previously presented materials.

4. *Attention Span*—Focusing on a task over time.

5. *Initiation of Activity*—Starting a physical or mental activity.

6. *Termination of Activity*—Stopping an activity at an appropriate time.

7. *Memory*—Recalling information after brief or long periods of time.

8. *Sequencing*—Placing information, concepts, and actions in order.

9. *Categorization*—Identifying similarities of and differences among pieces of environmental information.

10. *Concept Formation*—Organizing a variety of information to form thoughts and ideas.

11. *Spatial Operations*—Mentally manipulating the position of objects in various relationships.

12. *Problem Solving*—Recognizing a problem, defining a problem, identifying alterna-

tive plans, selecting a plan, organizing steps in a plan, implementing a plan, and evaluating the outcome.

13. *Learning*—Acquiring new concepts and behaviors.

14. *Generalization*—Applying previously learned concepts and behaviors to a variety of new situations.

C. *Psychosocial Skills and Psychological Components*—The ability to interact in society and to process emotions.

1. *Psychological*

a. *Values*—Identifying ideas or beliefs that are important to self and others.

b. *Interests*—Identifying mental or physical activities that create pleasure and maintain attention.

c. *Self-Concept*—Developing the value of the physical, emotional, and sexual self.

2. *Social*

a. *Role Performance*—Identifying, maintaining, and balancing functions one assumes or acquires in society (e.g., worker, student, parent, friend, religious participant).

b. *Social Conduct*—Interacting by using manners, personal space, eye contact, gestures, active listening, and self-expression appropriate to one's environment.

c. *Interpersonal Skills*—Using verbal and non-verbal communication to interact in a variety of settings.

d. *Self-Expression*—Using a variety of styles and skills to express thoughts, feelings, and needs.

3. *Self-Management*

a. *Coping Skills*—Identifying and managing stress and related factors.

b. *Time Management*—Planning and participating in a balance of self-care, work, leisure, and rest activities to promote satisfaction and health.

c. *Self-Control*—Modifying one's own behavior in response to environmental needs, demands, constraints, personal aspirations, and feedback from others.

III. Performance Contexts

Assessment of function in performance areas is greatly influenced by the contexts in which the individual must perform. Occupational therapy practitioners consider performance contexts when determining feasibility and appropriateness of interventions. Occupational therapy practitioners may choose interventions based on an understanding of contexts, or may choose interventions directly aimed at altering the contexts to improve performance.

A. *Temporal Aspects*

1. *Chronological*—Individual's age.

2. *Developmental*—Stage or phase of maturation.

3. *Life cycle*—Place in important life phases, such as career cycle, parenting cycle, or educational process.

4. *Disability status*—Place in continuum of disability, such as acuteness of injury, chronicity of disability, or terminal nature of illness.

B. *Environment*

1. *Physical*—Nonhuman aspects of contexts. Includes the accessibility to and performance within environments having natural terrain, plants, animals, buildings, furniture, objects, tools, or devices.

2. *Social*—Availability and expectations of significant individuals, such as spouse, friends, and caregivers. Also includes larger social groups which are influential in establishing norms, role expectations, and social routines.

3. *Cultural*—Customs, beliefs, activity patterns, behavior standards, and expectations accepted by the society of which the individual is a member. Includes political aspects, such as laws that affect access to resources and affirm personal rights. Also includes opportunities for education, employment, and economic support.

References

American Occupational Therapy Association. (1979). *Occupational therapy product output reporting system and uniform terminology for reporting occupational therapy services.* Rockville, MD: Author.

American Occupational Therapy Association. (1989). Uniform terminology for occupational therapy—Second edition. *American Journal of Occupational Therapy, 43,* 808-815.

American Occupational Therapy Association. (1993). Association policies—Definition of occupational therapy practice for state regulation (Policy 5.3.1). *American Journal of Occupational Therapy, 47,* 1117-1121.

7—MR of Part B Intermediary Outpatient Occupational Therapy (OT) Bills

The following is criteria for MR of OT services. Intermediaries use the OT edits to assist the reviewer in conducting focused MR within the intermediary budgeted levels. They conduct focused review using other selection criteria which is determined to be effective. If they choose to use any of the diagnostic edits listed, they do not change the visits and/or duration parameters without approval from CO. They must conform to the MR requirements for all outpatient claims from rehabilitation agencies, SNFs, hospitals, and HHAs that provide OT in addition to home health services.

The bill types are:

- Hospital = 12X and 13X;
- SNF = 22X and 23X;
- HHA = 34X,
- Rehabilitation agency, public health agency or clinic = 74X; and
- CORF = 75X.

These criteria do not apply to OT services provided under a home health plan of care. The criteria for MR case selection are based on ICD-9-CM diagnoses, elapsed time from start of care (at the billing provider) and number of visits. (See Exhibit 1.)

Denial of a bill solely on the basis that it exceeds the criteria in the edits is prohibited.

The edits are only for assisting the intermediary in selecting bills to review or for paying bills if they meet Level I criteria. They do not provide automatic coverage up to these criteria. They neither guarantee minimum nor set maximum coverage limits.

7.1—Level I Review

OT edits have been developed for a number of diagnoses. The diagnoses were selected on the basis that, when linked with a recent date of onset, there is a high probability that Medicare patients with these diagnoses will require skilled OT. The edits do not specify every diagnosis which may require OT, and the fact that a given diagnosis does not appear in the edits does not create a pre-

Source: Health Care Financing Administration. Program Integrity Manual. *Chapter 6, Section 7. May be downloaded free of charge at www.hcfa.gov/pubforms/*

sumption that OT services are not necessary or are inappropriate. Intermediaries do not approve or deny claims at Level I for medical necessity. They pay claims that suspend or pass the edits in Exhibit 1 without being subjected to Level II MR. However, they refer all claims which meet the focused MR criteria to Level II MR.

For patients receiving OT services only (V57.2) during an encounter/visit, providers list the appropriate V code for the service first, and, if documented, list the diagnosis or problem for which the services are performed second. The intermediary standard system must be programmed to read the diagnosis or problem listed second to determine if it meets the Level 1 OT edits.

EXAMPLE: Outpatient rehabilitation services, V57.2, for a patient with multiple sclerosis, 340.

The V code will be listed first, followed by the code for multiple sclerosis (V57.2, 340). Intermediaries must edit for multiple sclerosis not the V code. They use this same procedure for V57.81 (Orthotic training) V57.89 (Other) and V57.9 (Unspecified rehabilitation procedure).

The provider must submit the following information on the claim and the intermediary must evaluate bills at Level I based upon:

Facility and Patient Identification	Facility name, patient name, provider number, HICN, age.
Diagnosis	List the primary diagnosis for which OT services were furnished by ICD-9-CM code first. List other Dx(s) applicable to the patient or that influence care second.
Duration	The total length of time OT services have been furnished (in days) from the date treatment was initiated for the diagnosis being treated at the billing provider (including the last day in the current billing period).
Number of Visits	The total number of patient visits completed since OT services were initiated for the diagnosis being treated by the billing provider. The total visits to date (including the last visit in the billing period) must be given rather than for each separate bill (value code 51).
Date Treatment Started (Occurrence Code 44)	The date OT services were initiated by the billing provider for the primary medical Dx for which OT services are furnished.
Billing Period	When OT services began and ended in the billing period (from/through dates).

7.2—Level II Review Process

If a bill is selected for focused or intensified review, intermediaries refer it to the Level II health professional MR staff. If possible, they have occupational therapists review OT bills.

Once the bill is selected for focused MR, they review it in conjunction with the medical information submitted by the provider.

A—Payable OT Services

Intermediaries reimburse OT services only if they meet all requirements established by the Medicare guidelines and regulations. Each bill for OT services that is subjected to Level II MR must be supported with adequate medical documentation for the reviewer to make a determination. (For additional requirements see MIM §§3101.9 and 3148.)

7.3—MR Documentation

When a claim is referred to Level II review, intermediaries use the following pertinent data elements in addition to those used for Level I review.

Medical History	Obtain only the medical history which is pertinent to, or influences the OT treatment rendered, including a brief description of the functional status of the patient prior to the onset of the condition requiring OT, and any pertinent prior OT treatment.
Date of Onset (Occurrence Code 11)	The date of onset or exacerbation of the primary medical diagnosis for which OT services are being rendered by the billing provider.
Physician Referral and Date	
OT Initial Evaluation and Date	
Plan of Treatment Established	
Date of Last Certification	Obtain the date on which the plan of treatment was last certified by the physician.
Progress Notes	Obtain updated patient status reports concerning the patient's current functional abilities/limitations.

The following explains specific Level II documentation principles:

7.3.1—Medical History

If a history of previous OT treatment is not available, the provider supplies a general summary regarding the patient's past relevant medical history recorded during the initial evaluation with the patient/family or through contact with the referring physician. Information regarding prior OT treatment for the current condition, progress made, and treatment by the referring physician is provided when available. The level of function prior to the current exacerbation or onset is described.

The patient's medical history as it relates to OT, includes the date of onset and/or exacerbation of the illness or injury. If the patient has had prior therapy for the same condition, use that history in conjunction with the patient's current assessment to establish whether additional treatment is reasonable.

The history of treatments from a previous provider is necessary for patients who have transferred to a new provider. For example, if surgery has been performed, obtain the type and date. The date of onset and type of surgical procedure should be specific for diagnoses such as fractures. For other diagnoses, such as arthritis, the date of onset may be general. Establish it from the date the patient first required medical treatment. For other types of chronic diagnoses, the history gives the date of the change or deterioration in the patient's condition and a description of the changes that necessitate skilled OT.

7.3.2—Evaluation

Intermediaries approve an OT initial evaluation, (excluding routine screening) when it is reasonable and necessary for the therapist to determine if there is an expectation that either restorative or maintenance services are appropriate. They approve reevaluations when the patient exhibits a demonstrable change in physical functional ability, requiring reestablishment of appropriate treatment goals, or when reasonable and necessary, for ongoing assessment of the patient's rehabilitation needs. They approve initial evaluations or reevaluations that are reasonable and necessary based on the patient's condition, even though the expectations are not realized, or when the evaluation determines that skilled rehabilitation is not needed.

The OT evaluation establishes the physical and cognitive baseline data necessary for assessing expected rehabilitation potential, setting realistic goals, and measuring progress. The evaluation of the patient's functional deficits and level of assistance needed forms the basis for the OT goals. Objective tests and measurements are used (when possible) to establish base-line data.

The provider documents the patient's functional loss and the level of assistance requiring skilled OT intervention resulting from conditions such as those listed below.

A—Activities of Daily Living (ADL) Dependence

The individual is dependent upon skilled intervention for performance of activities of daily living. These include, but are not limited to, significant physical and/or cognitive functional loss, or loss of previous functional gains in the ability to:

- Feed, eat, drink;
- Bathe;
- Dress;
- Perform personal hygiene;
- Groom; or
- Perform toileting.

This could include management and care of orthoses and/or adaptive equipment, or customized therapeutic adaptations.

B—Functional Limitation

The individual is dependent upon skilled OT intervention in functional training, observation, assessment, and environmental adaptation due, but not limited to:

- Lack of awareness of sensory cues, or safety hazards;
- Impaired attention span;
- Impaired strength;
- In-coordination;
- Abnormal muscle tone;
- Range of motion limitations;
- Impaired body scheme;
- Perceptual deficits;
- Impaired balance/head control; and
- Environmental barriers.

C—Safety Dependence/Secondary Complications

A safety problem exists when a patient, without skilled OT intervention, cannot handle him/herself in a manner that is physically and/or cognitively safe. This may extend to daily living or to acquired secondary complications which could potentially intensify medical sequelae such as fracture nonunion, or skin breakdown. Safety dependence may be demonstrated by high probability of falling, lack of environmental safety awareness, swallowing difficulties, abnormal aggressive/destructive behavior, severe pain, loss of skin sensation, progressive joint contracture, and joint protection/preservation requiring skilled OT intervention to protect the patient from further medical complication(s).

If the goal is to increase the patient's functional abilities and decrease the level of assistance needed, the initial evaluation must measure the patient's starting functional abilities and level of assistance required.

7.3.3—Plan of Treatment

The OT plan of treatment must include specific functional goals and a reasonable estimate of when they will be reached (e.g., 6 weeks). It is not adequate to estimate "1 to 2 months on an ongoing basis." The provider submits changes in the plan with the progress notes. The plan must include the following information.

Type of OT Procedures	Describes the specific nature of the therapy to be provided.
Frequency of Visits	An estimate of the frequency of treatment to be rendered (e.g., 3x week). The provider's medical documentation should justify the intensity of services rendered. This is crucial when they are given more frequently than 3 times a week.
Estimated Duration	Identifies the length of time over which the services are to be rendered in days, weeks, or months.
Diagnoses	Includes the OT diagnosis if different from the medical diagnosis. The OT diagnosis should be based on objective tests, whenever possible.
Functional OT Goals (short- or long-term)	Reflects the occupational therapist's and/or physician's description of what functional physical/cognitive abilities the patient is expected to achieve. Assume that factors may change or influence the level of achievement. If this occurs, the occupational therapist or physician explains the factors which led to the change in functional goal(s).
Rehabilitation Potential	The occupational therapist's and/or physician's expectation concerning the patient's ability to meet the established goals.

7.3.4—Progress Reports

Progress reports or treatment summary for the billing period is used by the provider to document and report the following information:

- The patient's initial functional status;
- The patient's functional status and progress (or lack thereof) specific for this reporting period; including clinical findings (amount of physical and/or cognitive assistance needed, range of motion, muscle strength, unaffected limb measurements, etc.); and
- The patient's expected rehabilitation potential.

Where a valid expectation of improvement exists, the services are covered even though the expectation may not be realized. However, in such instances, the OT services are covered only to the time that no further significant practical improvement can be expected. Progress reports or status summaries must document a continued expectation that the patient's condition will continue to improve significantly in a reasonable and generally predictable period of time.

"Significant," means a generally measurable and substantial increase in the patient's present level of functional independence and competence, compared to that when treatment was initiated. Intermediaries should not interpret the term "signficant" so stringently that they deny a claim simply because of a temporary setback in the patient's progress. For example, a patient may experience an intervening medical complication or a brief period when lack of progress occurs. The medical reviewer may approve the claim if there is still a reasonable expectation that significant improvement in the patient's **overall safety or functional ability** will occur.

However, the provider should document the lack of progress and justify the need for continued skilled OT.

The provider must provide treatment information regarding the status of the patient during the billing period. The provider's progress notes and any needed reevaluation(s) must update the baseline information provided at the initial evaluation. If there is a change in the plan of treatment, it must be documented. Additionally, when a patient is continued from one billing period to another, the progress report(s) must reflect the comparisons between the patient's current functional status and that during the previous billing and/or initial evaluation.

Intermediaries conduct a MR of claims with an understanding that skilled intervention may be needed, and improvement in a patient's condition may occur, even where a patient's full or partial recovery is **not** possible. For example, a terminally ill patient may begin to exhibit ADL, mobility and/or safety dependence requiring OT. The fact that full or partial recovery is not possible or rehabilitation potential is not present, does not affect MR coverage decisions. The deciding factor is whether the services are considered reasonable, effective, treatment for the patient's condition and they require the skills of an occupational therapist, or whether they can be safely and effectively carried out by non-skilled personnel. The reasons for OT must be clear, as well as its goals, prior to a favorable coverage determination. They often require Level III review.

It is essential that the provider documents the updated status in a clear, concise, and objective manner. Objective tests and measurements are stressed when they are practical. The occupational therapist selects the method to demonstrate current patient status. However, the method chosen, as well as the measures used, should be consistent during the treatment duration. If the method used is changed, the reasons for the change should be documented, including how the new method relates to the old. The reviewer must have an overview of the purpose of treatment goals in order to compare the patient's current functional status to that in previous reporting periods.

Documentation of the patient's current functional status and level of assistance required compared to previous reporting period(s) is of paramount importance. The deficits in functional ability should be clear. Occupational therapists must document functional improvements (or lack thereof) as a result of their treatments. Documentation of functional progress must be stated in objective, measurable terms. The following illustrate these principles and demonstrate that significant changes may occur in one or more of the assistance levels:

7.3.4.1—Change in Level of Assistance

Occupational therapist's document assistance levels by describing the relationship between functional activities and the need for assistance. Within the assistance levels of minimum, moderate, and maximum there are intermediate gradations of improvement based on changes in behavior and response to assistance. **Improvements at each level must be documented** to compare the current cognitive and/or physical level achieved to that previously achieved.

While cognitive assistance often is the more severe and persistent disability, physical assistance often is the major obstacle to successful outcomes and subsequent discharge. Intermediaries should interpret the levels as follows:

A—Total Assistance

Total assistance is the need for 100 percent assistance by one or more persons to perform all physical activities and/or cognitive assistance to elicit a functional response to an external stimulation. An individual requires total assistance if the documentation indicates the patient is only able to initiate minimal voluntary motor actions and requires the skill of an occupational therapist to develop a therapeutic program or implement a maintenance program to prevent, or minimize, deterioration.

A cognitively impaired patient requires total assistance when documentation shows external stimuli are required to elicit automatic actions such as swallowing or responding to auditory stimuli. Skills of an occupational therapist are needed to identify and apply strategies for eliciting appropriate, consistent automatic responses to external stimuli.

B—Maximum Assistance

Maximum assistance is the need for 75 percent assistance by one person to physically perform any part of a functional activity and/or cognitive assistance to perform gross motor actions in response to direction. Patients require such assistance if maximum OT physical support and proprioceptive stimulation is needed for performance of each step of a functional activity, every time it is performed. A cognitively impaired patient, at this level, may need proprioceptive stimulation and/or one-to-one demonstration by the occupational therapist due to the patient's lack of cognitive awareness of other people or objects.

C—Moderate Assistance

Moderate assistance is the need for 50 percent assistance by one person to perform physical activities or constant cognitive assistance to sustain/complete simple, repetitive activities safely. A physically impaired patient requires moderate assistance if documentation indicates that moderate OT physical support and proprioceptive stimulation is needed each time to perform a functional activity.

The records submitted should state how a cognitively impaired patient requires intermittent one-to-one demonstration or intermittent cueing (physical or verbal) throughout the activity. Moderate assistance is needed when the occupational therapist/care-giver needs to be in the immediate environment to progress the patient through a sequence to complete an activity. This level of assistance is required to halt continued repetition of a task and to prevent unsafe, erratic or unpredictable actions that interfere with appropriate sequencing.

D—Minimum Assistance

Minimum assistance is the need for 25 percent assistance by one person for physical activities and/or periodic, cognitive assistance to perform functional activities safely. A physically impaired patient requires minimum assistance if documentation indicates that activities can only be performed after physical set-up by the occupational therapist or care-giver, and if physical help is needed to initiate, or sustain an activity. A review of alternate procedures, sequences and methods may be required. A cognitively impaired patient requires minimal assistance if documentation indicates help is needed in performing known activities to correct repeated mistakes, to check for compliance with established safety procedures, or to solve problems posed by unexpected hazards.

E—Standby Assistance

Standby assistance is the need for supervision by one person for the patient to perform new procedures adapted by the therapist for safe and effective performance. A patient requires such assistance when errors are demonstrated or the need for safety precautions are not always anticipated by the patient.

F—Independent Status

Independent status means that no physical or cognitive assistance is required to perform functional activities. Patients at this level are able to implement the selected courses of action, demonstrate lack of errors and anticipate safety hazards in familiar and new situations.

7.3.4.2—Change in Response to Treatment Within Each Level of Assistance

Significant improvement must be indicated by documenting a change in one or more of the following categories of patient responses:

A—Refusals

The patient may respond by refusing to attempt an activity because of fear or pain. The documentation should indicate the activity refused, the reasons, and how the OT plan addresses them. These responses are often secondary to a change in medical status or medications. If the refusals continue over several days, the therapy program should be put on "hold" until the patient is willing to attempt functional activities.

For the cognitively impaired patient, refusal to perform an activity can escalate into aggressive, destructive or verbally abusive behavior if the therapist or care-giver presses the patient to perform. In these cases, a reduction in these behaviors is considered significant progress, but must be documented, including the skilled OT provided to reduce the abnormal behavior.

For the psychiatrically impaired patient, refusals to participate in an activity frequently are symptoms of the diagnosis. The patient should not be put on a "hold" status due to refusals. If the documentation indicates that the patient is receiving OT, is contacted regularly, and is actively encouraged to participate, intermediaries medically review the claim to determine if reasonable and necessary skilled care has been rendered.

B—Inconsistency

The patient may respond by inconsistently performing functional tasks from day-to-day or within a treatment session. Intermediaries approve the claim when the documentation indicates a significant progression in consistency of performance of functional tasks within the same level of assistance.

C—Generalization

The patient may respond by applying previously learned concepts for performing an activity to another, similar activity. The records submitted should document a significant increase in scope of activities that the patient can perform, their type, and the skilled OT services rendered.

Examples of a new skilled functional activity are:

- Adding teaching of lower body dressing to a current program of upper body dressing;

- Increasing the ability to perform personal hygiene activities for health and social acceptance.

Examples of a new skilled compensatory technique (with or without adapted equipment) are:

- Teaching a patient techniques such as one-handed shoe tying;

- Teaching the use of a button hook for buttoning shirt buttons.

The acceptable length of time in treatment for various disorders is determined by the patient's documented functional abilities and progress.

7.3.5—Level of Complexity of Treatment

Intermediaries base decisions on the level of complexity of the services rendered by the occupational therapist and not what the patient is asked to do.

A—Skilled OT

The documentation must indicate that the severity of the physical, emotional, perceptual, or cognitive disability requires complex and sophisticated knowledge to identify current and potential capabilities. In addition, intermediaries consider instructions required by the patient and/or the patient's care-givers. Instructions may be required for activities that most healthy people take for granted. The special knowledge of an occupational therapist is required to decrease or eliminate limitations in functional activity performance. Occupational therapists must often address underlying factors which interfere with specific activities. These factors could be cognitive, sensory, or perceptual deficits.

The occupational therapist modifies the specific activity by using adapted equipment, making changes in the environment, altering procedures for accomplishing the task, and providing specialized assistance to meet the patient's current and potential abilities. Skilled services include, but are not limited to reasonable and necessary:

- Patient evaluations;
- Determinations of effective goals and services with the patient and patient's caregivers and other medical professionals;
- Analyzing and modifying functional tasks;
- Determination that the modified task obtains optimum performance through tests and measurements;
- Providing instructions of the task(s) to the patient, family, care-givers; and
- Periodically reevaluating the patient's status with corresponding readjustment of the OT program.

A period of practice may be approved for the patient and/or patient's care-givers to learn the steps of the task, to verify the task's effectiveness in improving function, and to check for safe and consistent performance.

B—Non-skilled OT

When the documentation indicates a patient has attained the therapy goals or has reached the point where no further significant improvement can be expected, the skills of an occupational therapist are not required to maintain function at the level to which it has been restored.

Examples of maintenance procedures:

- Daily feeding programs after the adapted procedures are in place;
- Routine exercise and strengthening programs;
- The practice of coordination and self-care skills on a daily basis; and
- Presenting information on energy conservation or pacing, but not having the patient perform the activity.

The intermediary may approve a claim because the patient requires the judgment and skills of the occupational therapist to design a safe and effective maintenance program and make periodic checks of its effectiveness. The services of an occupational therapist in carrying out the established maintenance program are not reasonable and necessary for the treatment of illness or injury and may not be approved.

7.3.6—Reporting on New Episode or Condition

Occasionally, a patient who is receiving or who has received OT services experiences a new illness. The provider must document the significance of any change to the patient's functional capabilities. This may be through pre and post episodic nursing notes or physician reports. If the patient is receiving treatment, it might be lengthened. If the patient had completed treatment a significant change in the patient's functional status must be documented to warrant a new treatment plan.

7.4—Other MR Considerations

A—Pain

Intermediaries consider documentation describing the presence or absence of pain and its effect on the patient's functional abilities in MR decisions. A description of its intensity, type, changing pattern, and location at specific joint ranges of motion materially aids correct decisions. Documentation should describe the limitations placed upon the patient's ADL, mobility and/or safety, as well as the subjective progress made in the reduction of pain through treatment.

B—Therapeutic Programs

The objective documentation should support the skilled nature of the program, and/or the need for the design and establishment of a maintenance OT program. The goals should be to increase functional abilities in ADL, mobility or patient safety. Documentation should indicate the goals and type of program provided.

Intermediaries may approve claims when the therapeutic program, because of documented medical complications, the condition of the patient, or complexity of the OT employed, must be rendered by, or under, the supervision of an occupational therapist. For example, while functional ADL may be performed safely and effectively by non-skilled personnel, fracture nonunion, severe joint pain, or other medical or safety complications may warrant skilled occupational therapist intervention to render the service and/or to establish a safe maintenance program. In these cases, the complications and the skilled services they require, must be documented by physician orders and/or dependencies in ADL, mobility and safety must be documented. The possibility of adverse effects from the improper performance of an otherwise unskilled service does not make it a skilled service unless documentation supports why skilled OT is needed for the patient's medical condition and/or safety.

Intermediaries approve the establishment and design of a maintenance exercise program to fit the patient's level of ADL, function, and any instructions to supportive personnel and/or family members need to safely and effectively carry it out. They may approve reevaluation when reasonable and necessary to readjust the maintenance program to meet the changing needs of the patient. There must be justification for readjusting a maintenance program, e.g., loss of previous functional gains.

C—Cardiac Rehabilitation Exercise

Occupational therapy is not covered when furnished in connection with cardiac rehabilitation exercise program services (see Coverage Issues Manual 35-25) unless there is also a diagnosed non-cardiac condition requiring it, e.g., a patient who is recuperating from an acute phase of heart disease may have had a stroke which requires OT. (While the cardiac rehabilitation exercise program may be considered by some a form of OT, it is a specialized program conducted and/or supervised by specially trained personnel whose services are performed under the direct supervision of a physician.)

D—Transfer Training

The documentation should describe the patient's functional limitations in transfer ability that warrant skilled OT intervention. Documentation includes the special transfer training needed to perform functional daily living skills and any training needed by supportive personnel and/or family members to safely and effectively carry it out. Intermediaries approve transfer training when the documentation supports a skilled need for evaluation, design and effective monitoring and instruction of the special transfer technique for safety and completion of the activities of daily living or mobility.

Documentation that supports only repetitious carrying out of the transfer method once established, and monitored for safety and completion does not show covered care.

E—Fabrication of and Training in Use of Orthoses, Prostheses and Adaptive Equipment

Intermediaries approve reasonable and necessary fabrication of orthoses, prostheses, adaptive equipment, and reasonable and necessary skilled training needed in their safe and effective use, if documentation indicates the need for the device and training in its use.

F—OT Forms

Documentation may be submitted on a specific form the intermediary requires or may be copies of the provider's record. However, the form must capture the needed MR information. If the reviewer chooses to require a particular form, show the OMB clearance number. The information submitted must be complete. If it is not, intermediaries return the bill for the additional information. The information required to review the bill is that which is required by an occupational therapist to properly treat a patient.

G—Certification and Re-certification

OT services must be certified and re-certified by a physician and must be furnished while the patient is under the care of a physician. OT services must be furnished under a written plan of treatment established by the physician or a qualified occupational therapist. If the plan is established by an occupational therapist, it must be reviewed periodically by the physician.

The plan of treatment must be established (reduced to writing by either professional or the provider when it makes a written record of oral orders) before treatment is begun. When outpatient OT services are continued under the same plan of treatment for a period of time, the physician must certify at least at 30-day intervals that there is a continuing need for them. Intermediaries obtain the re-certification when reviewing the plan of treatment since the same interval of at least 30 days is required for review of the plans. A re-certification must be signed by the physician, who reviewed the plan of treatment. Any changes to the treatment plan established by the occupational therapist must be in writing and signed by the therapist or by the attending physician. The physician may change a plan of treatment established by the occupational therapist. However, the occupational therapist may not alter a plan of treatment established by a physician.

7.4.1—Occupational Therapy Availability

Two or more disciplines may provide therapy services to the same patient. There may also be occasions where these services are duplicated. In many instances, the description of the services appears duplicated, but the documentation proves that they are not. Some examples where there is not a duplication include:

A—Transfers

PT instructs the patient in transfers to achieve the level of safety with the techniques. OT utilizes transfers as they relate to the performance of daily living skills (e.g., transfer from wheelchair to bathtub).

B—Pulmonary

PT instructs the patient in an adapted breathing technique. OT carries the breathing retraining into activities of daily living.

C—Hip Fractures/Arthroplasties

PT instructs the patient in hip precautions and gait training. OT reinforces the training with precautions for activities of daily living, e.g., lower extremity dressing, toileting, and bathing.

D—CVA

PT utilizes upper extremity neurodevelopmental (NDT) techniques to assist the patient in positioning the upper extremities on a walker and in gait training. PT utilizes NDT techniques to increase the functional use of the upper extremity for dressing, bathing, grooming, etc.

7.5—Focused MR Analysis

The HCFA edits may assist the intermediary in identifying OT claims for focused MR. Intermediaries perform regular evaluations of provider claims which pass or fail the edits. They must change the focused review claims selection based on the results of the evaluation. For example, a provider with an aberrant billing rate consistently just below the edit parameters is subject to intensified review. They develop procedures for focused MR based on each of the following trends or characteristics:

- Edits with high charges per aggregate bill charges;
- Providers billing a higher than average utilization of specific diagnostic codes that fall just below the edit parameters; and
- Specific principal DX codes, such as those with longer visits and duration; those representing the most frequent denials in pre-pay MR; special codes, e.g., 585, Chronic Renal Failure; 733.1, Senile Osteoporosis; and 290.0-290.9, Senile and Presenile Organic Psychotic Conditions; and/or certain edit groups such as 17, 19, and 29 in one quarter and others in the next quarter.

7.6—Outpatient Occupational Therapy Edits

The following edits do not represent normative (or average) treatment. It is prohibited to deny a bill solely on the basis that it exceeds the edits. The edits are for selecting bills for Level II MR.

EDIT IDENTIFICATION NUMBER	DIAGNOSIS	ICD-9-CM	NUMBER OF VISITS	DURATION (DAYS)
1	Neoplasms:			
	Bone and articular cartilage	170.0-170.3	16	48
	Connective tissue	171.0-171.2		
	Female breast	174.0-174.9 198.81		
	Bone or breast, NOS	239.2-239.3		
	Brain and nervous system	191.0-192-9		
	Hodgkin's Disease	201.0-201.9		
	Multiple myeloma	203.0-203.8		
	Leukemia	204.0-208.9		
	Brain and spinal cord; and nervous system	237.5-237.9		

EDIT IDENTIFICATION NUMBER	DIAGNOSIS	ICD-9-CM	NUMBER OF VISITS	DURATION (DAYS)
	Bone and articular cartilage, upper limb	170.4-170.5	24	62
	Brain and nervous system	225.0-225.9 239.6		
2	Schizophrenic disorder	295.30 thru 295.45 295.80-295.95	13	31
	Affective psychosis	296.00-296.99		
3	Parkinson's Disease	332.0-332.1	13	38
4	Meningitis/Encephalitis	320.0-323.9	16	62
	Intracranial and intraspinal abcess	324.0-324.9		
	Other extrapyramidal disease	333.0		
	Hydrocephalus and other cerebral	331.3-331.7		
	Degeneration	331.89		
	Huntington's Chorea and other choreas	333.4-333.9		
	Spinocerebellar disease	334.0-334.9		
	ALS and other motor neuron diseases	335.20-335.9		
	Other diseases of the spinal cord Unspecified disorder of autonomic N.S.	336.0-336.9		
	Multiple Sclerosis	337.9		
	Demyelinating Diseases of CNS			
	Hemiplegia (old unspecified)	340		
	Other unspecified disorders of nervous system	341.8-341.9 342.0-342.9		
	Infantile cerebral palsy			
	Late effects of CVA	349.0-349.9		
	Other conditions of brain	343.0-343.9		

EDIT IDENTIFICATION NUMBER	DIAGNOSIS	ICD-9-CM	NUMBER OF VISITS	DURATION (DAYS)
	Other ill defined cerebrovascular diseases	438 348.0-348.9		
	Intracranial injury	437.0-437.9 851.00-854.19		
5	Cerebral hemorrhage, occlusion, stenosis	430-434.9	28	72
	CVA, acute	436		
	Concussion, Loss of consciousness Without return to previous level	850.4		
	Intracranial injury including those with skull Fx	800.70-800.99 801.70-801.99 803.20-803.49 803.70-803.99 804.70-804.99 800.30-800.49 801.49 804.20-804.49		
6	Other paralytic syndromes, paraplegia Quadriplegia	344.0-344.9	32	93
7	Late effects polio	138	13	40
	Disorders of peripheral nerves	353.0-356.9 357.1-359.9	16	62
	Fx of vertebral column	806.00-806.5	30	93
	with spinal cord injury	952.00-953.1	24	62
	without spinal bone	953.4		
	injury	953.8		
	Peripheral nerve injury	955.0-955.9 957.0-957.9		
	Acute infective polyneuritis	357.0		
	Disturbance of skin	782.0	12	38

EDIT IDENTIFICATION NUMBER	DIAGNOSIS	ICD-9-CM	NUMBER OF VISITS	DURATION (DAYS)
8	Diabetes with peripheral circulatory disorders	250.00-250.01 250.60-250.711662		
	Diseases of circulatory system	402.0-429.9	12	38
	Postmastectomy lymphedema other lymphedema	457.0-457.1	10	31
9	Chronic ulcer of skin	707.0-707.9	12	31
	Diabetes, ulcer (skin)	250.80-250.81		
	Cellulitis, finger	681.00-681.02		
	Open wounds	880.00-884.2		
	Burns (second degree)	941.20-941.29 942.20-942.29 943.20-943.29 944.20-944.28 946.2 & 949.2	12	18
10	Emphysema, asthma Chronic airway obstruction	492.0-493.91 496	8	31
11	Chronic renal failure	585	12	38
	Acute renal failure	584.9		
	Nephritis, nephropathy	583.9		
	Renal failure unspecified	586		
12	Lupus erythematosus	695.4	16	62
	Diffuse disease of connective tissue	710.0-710.9		
	Arthropathy associated with infection	711.00-711.59		
	Rheumatoid arthritis and inflammatory polyarthropathies	714.0-714.9		
	Gouty arthopathy	274.0		
13	Osteoarthrosis and allied disorders	715.00-716.99	13	31

EDIT IDENTIFICATION NUMBER	DIAGNOSIS	ICD-9-CM	NUMBER OF VISITS	DURATION (DAYS)
14	Internal derangement of joint, other derangement of joint and other unspecified disorders of joint	718.00-718.99	16	48
15	Dorsopathies	720.0-722.0 723.0 723.3- 723.4 723.9	13	31
	Osteitis deformans	731.0		
	Aseptic necrosis	733.40-733.41		
	Disorder of bone and cartilage	733.81-733.99		
	Other acquired deformities	738.8-738.9		
	Other and unspecified anomalies of musculoskeletal system	756.9		
	Osteomyelitis	730.00-730.29		
	Acquired deformities	736.00-736.89</TD		
	Pathological Fx	733.1	12	31
16	Peripheral enthesopathies and allied syndromes	725-726.4 726.8-727.05	1331	
	Disorders of muscles, tendons, their attachments and other soft tissues	727.2-727.50 727.59-727.64 727.69 727.81-728.6 728.81-729.2 729.39-729.9		
17	Senile dementia	290.0-290.9	10	31
	Other cerebral degenerations	331.0-331.2 331.9		
	Malaise, fatigue	780.7		
	Syncope/collapse convulsions, dizziness	780.2-780.4		
	Other symptoms involving nervous and musculoskeletal system	781.9		
	Debility, unspecified and other	799.3 799.8-799.9		

EDIT IDENTIFICATION NUMBER	DIAGNOSIS	ICD-9-CM	NUMBER OF VISITS	DURATION (DAYS)
	Abnormal involuntary movements	781.0	12	38
	Incoordination, transient paralysis of limb T.I.A.	781.3-781.4 435.0-435.9	1338	
18	Fx of vertebral column without cord injury	805.00-805.9	13	38
	Fx of rib, sternum	807.00-807.4	12	38
	Fx of clavicle	810.00-810.03		
	Fx of unspecified bone	829.0-829.1		
19	Fx of pelvis Fx of femur	808.0-808.9 820.00-821.39	13	31
20	Fx of scapula	811.00-811.19	13	31
21	Fx of humerus Fx of radius and ulna, Fx of carpals, Fx of metacarpals and phalanges	812.00-819.1	22	62
	Dislocations Crushing injury	831.00-834.12 927.00-927.9 929.0-929.9	18	62
22	Sprains and strains	840.4-842.19	18	62
	Late effects of strains, sprains	905.6-905.7	13	31
	Dislocations, Contusions	923.3-923.9		
	Injury, other and unspecified	959.2-959.5		
23	Amputation upper	885.0-887.7	32	93
	lower	897.0-897.7	12	38
24	Burns (3rd and 4th degree)	941.30-941.59 942.30-942.55 942.59 943.30-943.56 943.49 944.30-944.58 946.3-946.5 949.3-949.5		

EDIT IDENTIFICATION NUMBER	DIAGNOSIS	ICD-9-CM	NUMBER OF VISITS	DURATION (DAYS)
25	Joint replacement	V43.6	18	48
	Problem with limbs	V49.0-49.9	13	48
	Convalescence following FX	V66.4		
	Follow-up exam FX	V67.4		
	Fitting and adjustment of prosthetic device, Artificial arm Other	V52.0		
	Orthopedic aftercare involving removal internal fixation device	V54.0	1031	
	Observation for specified suspected condition	V71.8		
	Orthopedic aftercare	V54.8-V54.9	12	38
	Other aftercare following surgery	V58.4		
	Other specified aftercare	V58.8		
	Unspecified aftercare	V58.9		
	Other follow-up exam	V67.59-V67.9		
	Late effects Fx, spine and upper extremities	905.1-905.2	13	38
	Late effects tendon injury	905.8		
	Late effects traumatic amputation	905.9		
	Late effects of injuries	906.0-909.9		
	Complications of surgical and medical care	996.4 996.60-997.1 997.6-997.9 998.3 998.5 998.8-998.9 999.9		

EDIT IDENTIFICATION NUMBER	DIAGNOSIS	ICD-9-CM	NUMBER OF VISITS	DURATION (DAYS)
26	Malnutrition (moderate)	263.0	13	38
	protein/calorie	263.8-263.9		
	Abnormal weight loss	783.2		
	Feeding difficulties	783.3		
	Dysphagia	787.2		

8—Forms HCFA-700/701, Outpatient Rehabilitation Services Forms

The outpatient rehabilitation services forms, Forms HCFA-700/701, are combined medical review (MR), certification/re-certification plan of treatment (POT) forms for outpatient Part B, physical therapy (PT), occupational therapy (OT) and speech language pathology (ST). The forms' design promotes national consistency in reporting and reducing unnecessary requests for additional medical records. HCFA will not mandate use of the hard copy Forms HCFA 700/701. However, some providers have made significant investments in the use of these forms. Therefore, intermediaries must accept hard copy versions of the Forms HCFA-700/701 if the provider chooses to use them. Providers complete the Form HCFA-700 only for initial bills. For interim-to-discharge bills, the provider completes the Form HCFA-701.

Intermediaries use the forms as a source of supporting medical information. They request forms HCFA-700/701 when the reviewers need supporting medical information to help determine whether services are reasonable and necessary.

Intermediaries base payment and denial decisions on information contained in these forms. However, they request additional information when additional medical information is needed to support a decision. A denial determination may not be made solely on the reviewer's general inferences about beneficiaries with similar diagnoses or on data related to utilization.

Instead, reviewers must make determinations based upon clear objective clinical evidence concerning the beneficiary's unique medical condition and individual need for care.

They do not routinely require providers to submit the Forms HCFA-700/701. They request only the Form HCFA-700 for initial bills and obtain the Form HCFA-701 for subsequent bills. They obtain photocopies of prior months forms HCFA-700-701 only when needed for coverage determinations.

If the intermediary standard system can retrieve previously submitted Forms HCFA-700/701 information/data, intermediaries inform providers not to send copies.

Providers must complete all applicable items on the forms. However, if an item is blank and a coverage determination can be made, intermediaries should process the claim. Providers may complete items with "N/A," not applicable, when the item does not apply (e.g., no hospitalization occurred). If information is needed for a coverage decision in an item marked as "N/A" (or left blank), they request the information from the provider.

Intermediaries obtain completed forms HCFA-700/701 from acute hospitals, skilled nursing facilities (SNFs), home health agencies (HHAs), comprehensive outpatient rehabilitation facilities (CORFs), rehabilitation agencies, public health agencies, and clinics (bill types 12X, 13X, 22X, 23X, 34X, 74X, and 75X). They obtain a separate form for each therapy discipline (revenue code) billed.

For example, if a patient received treatment for two services (i.e., PT and OT), the provider must submit two forms. These forms may also be used for outpatient hospital cardiac rehabilitation (CR), respiratory therapy (RT), or psychiatric services (PS). CORFs may also use the forms for skilled nursing (SN) and medical social services.

8.1—Electronic Attachments

Providers submitting batch attachments must use the current version of the UB-92 flat file record type (RT) 77. This information may be sent with claim data or independent of claim data. See MIM Addenda A, B, and D and PIM Chapter 9§ for further instructions. Intermediaries require the provider to maintain the information to support the electronic format in the beneficiary's medical record, whether hard copy, or electronic. They request additional information to support a decision only as necessary.

8.1.1—Instructions for Completion of Form HCFA-700, Plan of Treatment for Outpatient Rehabilitation

The Provider submits the following information on the Form HCFA-700:

1	Patient's Name	This item indicates the patient's last name, first name, and middle initial as shown on the health insurance card.
2	Provider Number	This item indicates the six digit number issued by Medicare to the provider. The number contains two digits, a hyphen, and four digits (e.g., 00-7000).
3	HICN	This item indicates the numeric plus alpha indicator(s) as shown on the patient's health insurance card, certification award, utilization notice, temporary eligibility notice, or as reported by the SSO.
4	Provider Name	This item indicates the name of the Medicare billing provider.
5	Medical Record Number	This item indicates the patient's medical/clinical record number issued by the billing provider.
6	Onset Date	This item indicates either the onset date of the primary medical diagnosis (if it is a new diagnosis) or the date of the most recent exacerbation of a previous diagnosis. If the exact day is not known, "01" is used for the day (e.g., 020199). This date must match Occurrence Code 11 on the UB-92.
7	SOC (Start of Care) Date	This item indicates the six digit month, day, and year on which rehabilitation services began at the billing provider, i.e., MMDDYY (021599). **The SOC date is the first Medicare billable visit (normally the date of initial evaluation). This date remains the same on subsequent claims until the patient is discharged or the claim is denied.** A provider may suspend services and later resume them under the same SOC date in accordance with its internal procedures. The SOC date may also reflect a re-initiation after discharge or denial if for an exacerbation. For PT, the SOC date must correspond to Occurrence Code 35 on the UB-92, for OT code 44, for SLP code 45, and for CR code 46.
8	Type	The provider checks this item for the type of therapy furnished, i.e., PT, OT, SLP, for outpatient hospital CR, RT, or PS. CORFs may also check SN and/pr MSS (SW).

9	Primary Diagnosis	This item indicates the medical diagnosis (DX) that has resulted in the therapy disorder and which is most closely related to the current plan of care for therapy. The diagnosis may or may not be related to the patient's most recent hospital stay but must relate to the services furnished by the provider. If more than one diagnosis is treated concurrently, the provider enters the diagnosis that represents the most intensive services (over 50 percent of rehabilitation effort for the revenue code billed). The primary DX may change on subsequent forms if the patient develops an acute condition or an exacerbation of a secondary diagnosis requiring intensive services different than established on the initial plan of treatment (POT). In all such instances, the date treatment started at the billing provider remains the same until the patient is discharged.
10	Treatment Diagnosis	This item indicates the DX for which rehabilitative services were furnished (e.g., for SLP the treatment DX is a communication disorder). For example, while cerebrovascular accident (CVA) may be the primary medical DX, aphasia might be the SLP treatment DX. If the treatment DX is the same as the medical DX, the word "same" is used in this item.
11	Visits From Start of Care	This item indicates the cumulative total visits that were completed since the start of services at the billing provider for the treated DX through the last visit on the bill. This total corresponds to the UB-92 Value Code 50 for PT, 51 for OT, 52 for SLP, or 53 for CR.
12	Plan of Treatment Functional Goals	
	A. Functional goals	This item indicates the initial short and long-term goals in measurable, objective, and functional terms. Included are the functional levels (or safety levels) the patient is expected to achieve upon discharge as a result of therapy services. Also, indicated are the levels the patient is to achieve outside of the therapeutic environment. Time-oriented goals are entered when applicable. For example, communicate basic physical needs and emotional status within weeks (as functional goal for SLP).
	B. Plan	This item indicates the initial overall plan of care, type, and specific nature of rehabilitation procedures that are to be furnished (i.e., treatment the therapist is using: procedures or modalities used).
13	Signature	The signature (or name) and professional designation of the professional who established the plan of treatment is entered in this item. A qualified therapist or speech/language pathologist may establish the POT for PT, OT, or SLP.
14	Frequency	This item indicates the frequency of treatment the provider expects to furnish per day, week, or month. Also, projected is the length of time the provider expects to furnish services. This is to be expressed in days, weeks, or months (e.g., 3/Wk x 4 Wks).

15	Physician's Signature	The physician signs and dates this item if the Form HCFA-700 is to be used as the physician's certification. If you use an alternative signed certification form, the "On File" box should be checked (Item 18). Identify the period of certification in Item 17 on the HCFA-700. When certification is not required, the provider uses "N/A." Rubber signature stamps are not acceptable as the physician signature. The provider must keep the form containing the physician's original signature on file at the provider site.
16	Date	This item indicates the date the physician signed the form in 6 digits (i.e., month, day, and year).
17	Certification	This item indicates the six digit month, day, and year (i.e., MMDDYY 021599-041599) which identifies the period covered by the POT. The "From" date for the initial certification must match the SOC date. The "Through" date can be up to, but never exceed, 30 days (60 days for CORFs). The "Through" date is repeated on a subsequent recertification as the next sequential "From" date. Services delivered on the "Through" date are covered in the next re-certification period.
18	On File	This box is checked if the provider uses the form for certification. The provider is to enter the name of the physician who certified the POT that is on file at the billing provider. If certification is not required for the type of service checked in Item 8, the name of the physician who referred or ordered the service should be entered, but the "On File" box is not to be checked.
19	Prior Hospitalization	This item indicates the six digit month, day, and year (inclusive dates) of the most recent hospitalization that is pertinent to the patient's condition or primary DX billed (date from 1st day of admission through discharge day). The provider enters "N/A" if this is not applicable. If the period is not known, they enter "N/A."

20	Initial Assessment	This item indicates a brief historical narrative of the injury or illness and the reason(s) for referral as they relate to the primary or treatment DX. The providers use the following guidelines when constructing their narrative: Describe pertinent functional deficits and clinical findings and problems found on the initial assessment. Use objective, measurable terminology such as tests and measurements; Assess the patient's activities of daily living (ADL), range of motion (ROM), strength, functional abilities, psychological status, level of assistance required, and pertinent speech-language functional deficit findings. Include tests administered with scores; Relate pertinent safety precautions and medical complications which require skilled intervention that may affect a patient's progress or attainment of goals; List the patient's rehabilitation potential, cognitive status that affects functional ability, and psychological, respiratory, cardiac tests and measurements, as appropriate; and Document audio logic results, vision status, and use or status of amplification for patients receiving speech reading services.
21	Functional Level	This item indicates the patient's functional physical, cardiac, respiratory, or psychological status reached at the end of the claim period. The provider is to compare results to that shown on the initial assessment (Item 20). Record functional levels and progress in objective terminology. Include test results and measurements as appropriate. Record information about any change in functional level related to the goal(s) of treatment. When only a few visits have been made (e.g., evaluation) and when there is no change in function, the training/treatment furnished and the patient's response to the visit(s) are recorded. The provider checks the box titled "Continue Services" if services were continued. The provider checks the box titled "DC Services" if services were discontinued (e.g., if the patient was discharged).
22	Service Dates	This item indicates the "From/Through" dates that represent this billing period. If the provider uses this form for certification (with the exception of CORFs), this billing period should be monthly. The "From/Through" dates in field 22 on the UB-92 must match the dates in this item. Providers may not use "00" in the date, e.g., 042799 for April 27, 1999.

8.1.2—Instructions for Completion of Form HCFA-701, Updated Plan Progress for Outpatient Rehabilitation

Fields 1 through 11 are the same on forms HCFA 700 and HCFA 701. the provider submits the following information for the remaining fields on the Form HCFA-701:

Exhibits of form HCFA 700 and HCFA 701 can be found in Chapter (HCFA: NEED COPY OF FORM 700/701) of the PIM Manual.

12	Current Frequency Duration	This item indicates the frequency of treatment the provider expects to furnish per day, week or month. Also, projected is the length of time the services are expected to be furnished per days, weeks, or months (e.g., 3/Wk x 4Wks).
13	Current Plan Update, Functional Goals	This item indicates the functional treatment goals for the patient for this billing period. The provider is to state the goals in measurable, objective terms. They are to stress functional short-term goals to reach overall long-term outcomes that the patient is expected to achieve upon discharge (Item 12, HCFA-700). They are to document changes to the initial plan of treatment and effective date(s). providers must estimate time-frames to reach goals when possible. They are to record procedures or modalities used. If appropriate, they are to describe justification of intensity or any changes to the initial plan in Item 18.
14	Re-certification	This code indicates the six digit month, day, and year, i.e., MMDDYY (061598-071598), that identifies the period covered by the plan of treatment. The "From" date for the initial certification must match the SOC date. The "Through" date can be up to, but never exceed 30 days (60 days for CORFs). The provider is to repeat the "Through" date on a subsequent recertification as the next sequential "From" date. Services delivered on the "Through" date are covered in the next recertification period. On interim CORF claims, "N/A" is used.

EXAMPLE: Initial certification "From" date 051599. Initial certification "Through" date 061599. Re-certification "From" date 061599. Re-certification "Through" date 071599.
Certification/re-certification is **required for outpatient PT, OT, and SLP and CORF plans of care. Certification is required for partial hospitalization PS.** When certification/re-certification is not required, the provider uses "N/A."
There is no requirement that the provider enter the certification on the Forms HCFA-700/701 or handle it in any specific way as long as the reviewer can determine, where necessary, that certification/re-certification requirements are met.

15	Physician Signature	If the provider uses the Form HCFA-701 as the physician's recertification, the physician must sign and date the statements. If not, when appropriate, the "On File" box in Item 17 must be checked. Identify the period of recertification in Item 14 on the form. For interim CORF claims and when re-certification is not required, the provider must use the "N/A" box. If the physician established the plan of treatment, the physician must sign both Items 15 and 19. If the plan of treatment is established by a PT, OT, or speech-language pathologist, that therapist or speech-language pathologist must sign the plan (Item 19). A physician who has knowledge of the care signs the certification/re-certification.

16	Date	This item indicates the date the physician signs the certification/ re-certification in six digits (month, date, and year). The date must be shown even if the provider checks the "On File" box in Item 18.
17	On File	When the "On File" box is checked, request the certification/re-certification in accordance with your internal procedures, that are approved by your Regional Office (RO).
18	Reason(s) for Continuing Treatment This Billing Period	This item indicates the major reason(s) justifying continued therapy and the need for additional rehabilitation. Safety/medical complications are to be stated when further applicable. In the event of discharge, the provider is to provide the reason.
19	Signature	The professional who furnishes care or supervises services must enter his/her signature and professional designation.
20	Date	This item indicates the date of the signature in 6 digits (month, day, and year).
21	Continued or Discontinued	The provider checks this box to identify whether services are continued, or discontinued (last bill).
22	Functional Level (end of claim period)	This item indicates the functional level(s) and progress made at the end of the billing period. Obtain objective tests and measurements when practical. The providers are to date specific short-term gains when practical (e.g., when the patient is able to consistently perform them in this billing period). Providers are to document pertinent safety problems and/or precautions needed. They are to update the patient's current functional level(s) and progress (or lack of progress with an explanation) achieved as compared to the previous month and/or initial assessment. They are to document assistive devices used. Providers are to submit concise, quality, objective documentation and restrict subjective quantity. They should avoid such terms as "improved strength" or "improved communication." Providers billing 5 or more visits per week should use this space to update progress at 2 weeks and at the end of the claim period.
NOTE: When relating functional level(s) and progress made, the reviewer considers that a patient might not progress (or progress little) during a part of a claim period and the patient notes will reflect that fact. This should not be interpreted so stringently to result in an impulsive termination of coverage at that point. Medically review the entire period (including the prior month in relation to the full month in question) to determine coverage.		
23	Service Dates	This item indicates the "From and Through" dates which represent the billing period. If the provider uses the form for certification/re-certification, with the exception of CORFs, the provider bills monthly. The "From and Through" dates in field 23 are to match the dates on UB-92. Providers should not use "))" in the date, e.g., 042799 for April 27, 1999.

Medicare Fiscal Intermediaries

MEDICARE FISCAL INTERMEDIARIES BY STATE – PART A.		
Alabama	Mutual of Omaha	402-351-2860
Alaska	Premera Blue Cross	425-670-1010
American Samoa	Hawaii Medical Ser.	808-948-6247
Arizona	Blue Cross of Arizona	602-864-4298
Arkansas	BlueCross/Blue Shield	501-378-2173
California	Blue Cross of California	805-383-2038
Colorado	Blue Cross/Blue Shield	800-442-2620
Connecticut	United Health Care	203-639-3222
Delaware	Empire Medicare Ser.	800-442-8430
Florida	Blue Cross/Blue Shield	904-355-8899
Georgia	Blue Cross/Blue Shield	706-322-4082
Guam	Hawaii Medical Ser.	808-948-6247
Hawaii	Hawaii Medical Ser.	808-948-6247
Idaho	Blue Cross/Blue Shield/Oregon	503-721-7000
Illinois	Adminastar Federal	312-938-6266
Indiana	Adminastar Federal	800-622-4792
Iowa	Wellmark Blue Cross/Blue Shield of Iowa	712-279-8650
Kansas	Blue Cross/Blue Shield –Part A	800-445-7170
Kentucky	Adminastar Federal	800-999-7608
Louisiana	Trispan Health Services/Medicare	800-932-7644

MEDICARE FISCAL INTERMEDIARIES BY STATE – PART A.		
Maine	Assoc. Hospital Svc. of Maine	888-896-4997
Maryland	Trailblazers	800-444-4606
Massachusetts	Assoc. Hospital Svc. of Maine	888-896-4997
Michigan	Wisconsin United Govern. Ser.	313-225-8317
Minnesota	Blue Cross/Blue Shield	800-382-2000
Mississippi	Trispan Health Ser./Medicare	800-932-7644
Missouri	Trispan Health Ser. Medicare	800-932-7644
Montana	Blue Cross/Blue Shield	800-447-7828 Ext. 4086
Nebraska	Blue Cross/Blue Shield	401-390-1850
Nevada	Blue Cross of California	805-383-2038
New Hampshire/ Vermont	Health Service	603-695-7205
New Jersey	Horizon Blue Cross/Blue Shield of New Jersey	973-456-2112
New Mexico	Blue Cross/Blue Shield	800-442-2620
New York	Empire Medicare Ser.	800-442-8430
North Carolina	Blue Cross/Blue Shield	800-685-1512 In-state calls only
North Dakota	Meridian Mutual Insur. Company	800-247-2267
Northern Mariana Islands	Hawaii Medical Ser.	808-948-6247
Ohio	Adminastar Federal	513-852-4314
Oklahoma	Blue Cross/Blue Shield	918-560-3367
Oregon	Blue Cross/Blue Shield/Oregon	503-721-7000
Pennsylvania	Veritus Medicare Ser.	800-853-1419
Puerto Rico	Cooperativa DeSeguros DeVida	800-986-5656 In-state calls only
Rhode Island	Blue Cross/Blue Shield of Rhode Island	800-662-5157
South Carolina	Blue Cross/Blue Shield of South Carolina	803-788-4660
South Dakota	Wellmark	712-279-8650
Tennessee	Blue Cross/Blue Shield	423-755-5955
Texas	Blue Cross/Blue Shield	800-442-2620
Utah	Blue Cross/Blue Shield	801-333-2410

MEDICARE FISCAL INTERMEDIARIES BY STATE – PART A.		
New Hampshire/ Vermont	Health Service	603-695-7204
Virgin Islands	Cooperativa DeSeguros DeVida	800-986-5656 In-state calls only
Virginia	Blue Cross/Blue Shield	540-985-3931
Washington	Premera Blue Cross	425-670-1010
Washington, D.C.	Mutual of Omaha	402-351-2860
West Virginia	Blue Cross/Blue Shield	540-985-3931
Wisconsin	Blue Cross/Blue Shield of Wisconsin	414-224-4954
Wyoming	Blue Cross/Blue Shield	800-442-2376

MEDICARE FISCAL INTERMEDIARIES BY STATE – PART B		
Alabama	Blue Cross/Blue Shield	800-292-8855
Alaska	Noridian Mutual Insur. Company	800-444-4606
American Samoa	Noridian Mutual Insur. Company	800-444-4606
Arizona	Noridian Mutual Insur. Company	800-444-4606
Arkansas	Blue Cross/Blue Shield of Arkansas	800-482-5525 In-state calls only
California	Transamerica Occidental Life	800-675-2255 – Counties of Los Angeles, Orange, San Diego, Ventura, Imperial, San Luis Obispo, Santa Barbara, National Herigage Co. – 800-952-8627
Colorado	Noridian Mutual Insur. Company	800-332-6681
Connecticut	United Health Care	800-982-6819 In-state calls only
Delaware	Trailblazers	800-444-4606 Also services Fairfax & Alexandria Counties, Arlington, VA
Florida	Blue Cross/Blue Shield	800-333-7586 In-state calls only
Georgia	Cahara County Benefit Administration	800-737-0827
Guam	Noridian Mutual Insur. Company	800-444-4606
Hawaii	Noridian Mutual Insur. Company	800-444-4606
Idaho	Signa Medicare	800-342-8900 In-state calls only
Illinois	Wisconsin Physician's Service	800-642-6930
Indiana	Adminastar Federal	800-622-4792
Iowa	Noridian Mutual Insur. Company	800-532-1285
Kansas	Blue Cross/Blue Shield of Kansas	800-633-1133
Louisiana	Louisiana Medicare Part B	800-462-9666 In-state calls only
Kentucky	Adminastar Federal	800-999-7608
Massachusetts	National Heritage Insur. Co.	800-882-1228
Michigan	Wisconsin Physician's Service	800-482-4045

MEDICARE FISCAL INTERMEDIARIES BY STATE – PART B		
Minnesota	United Health Care	800-352-2762 In-state calls only
Mississippi	United Health Care	800-682-5417 In-state calls only
Missouri	Blue Cross/Blue Shield of Arkansas	800-392-3070 – St. Louis City and County, Jefferson County, and Area 99 Blue Cross/Blue Shield, 800-432-8216 – Out-of-State calls only – 800-432-0216 – out of state calls only – 800-892-5900 – in-state calls only
Montana	Blue Cross/Blue Shield of Montana	800-332-6146 In-state calls only
Nebraska	Blue Cross/Blue Shield	800-633-1113
Nevada	Noridian Mutual Insur. Company	800-444-4606
New Hampshire	National Heritage Insur. Company	800-882-1228
New Jersey	Empire Medicare Ser. – New Jersey Operations	800-462-9306
New Mexico	Blue Cross/Blue Shield of Arkansas	
New York	Blue Cross/Blue Shield	800-252-6550
Services Upstate New York	Empire Medicare Ser.	800-442-8430
Services Downstate New York	Group Health, Inc.	800-632-5572 – Queens County only
North Carolina	Signa Medicare	800-672-3071 In-state calls only
North Dakota	Meridian Mutual Insur. Company	800-247-2267
Northern Mariana Islands	Meridian Mutual Insur. Company	800-444-4606
Ohio	Nationwide Mutual Insur. Company	800-848-0106
Oklahoma	Blue Cross/Blue Shield of Arkansas	800-522-9079
Oregon	Meridian Mutual Insur. Company	800-442-4606
Pennsylvania	Xact Medicare Services	800-382-1274 In-state calls only
Puerto Rico	Triple and Inc.	800-474-7448 In-state calls only
Rhode Island	Blue Cross/Blue Shield of Rhode Island	800-662-5170

MEDICARE FISCAL INTERMEDIARIES BY STATE – PART B		
North Carolina	Palmeto Government Benefits Admin.	800-868-2522
North Dakota	Meridian Mutual Insur. Company	800-437-4762
Tennessee	Signa Medicare	800-342-8900 In-state calls only
Texas	Blue Cross/Blue Shield	800-442-2620
Utah	Blue Cross/Blue Shield	800-426-3477
Vermont	National Heritage Insur. Company	800-882-1228
Virgin Islands	Triple and Inc.	800-474-7448 In-state calls only
Virginia	Trailblazers	800-444-4606 – All services Fairfax and Alexandria Counties
Arlington Virginia	United Health Care/Travelers Insur.	800-552-3423 In-State calls only
Washington	Meridian Mutual Insur. Company	800-444-4606
Washington, D.C.	Trailblazers	800-444-4606 – Also services Fairfax and Alexandria Counties, Arlington Virginia
West Virginia	Nationwide Mutual Insur. Company	800-848-0106
Wisconsin	Wisconsin Physician's Service	800-944-0051 In-state calls only
Wyoming	Meridian Mutual Insur. Company	800-442-2371

Insurance Commissioners

STATE INSURANCE COMMISSIONERS		
Alabama	David Parsons, Acting Commissioner Alabama Dept. of Insur. 201 Monroe Street, Suite 1700 P.O. Box 303351 Montgomery, AL 36104	334-269-3550 Fax: 334-241-4192 E-mail: insdept@insurance.state.al.us Web site: www.aldoi.org

Alaska	Robert Lohr, Director
	Department of Community and
	    Economic Development
	Division of Insurance
	3601 C Street, Suite 1324
	Anchorage, AK 99503-5948
		907-269-7900
		Fax: 907-269-7910
		E-mail: insurance@dced.state.ak.us
		Web site: www.dced.state.ak.us/
		    insurance

	John Ference, Acting Deputy Director Department of Community and Economic Development Division of Insurance P.O. Box 110805 Juneau, AK 99811-0805 TDD/TTY: 907-465-5437	907-465-2515 Fax: 907-465-3422 E-mail: insurance@dced.state.ak.us Web site: www.commerce.state.ak.us
Arizona	Charles Cohen, Director Arizona Department of InsuranceT 2910 North 44th Street, Suite 210 Phoenix, AZ 85018-7256	602-912-8444 oll free in AZ: 1-800-325-2548 Fax: 602-954-7008 (complaints) Web site: www.state.az.us/id
Arkansas	Mike Pickens, Commissioner Arkansas Department of Insurance 1200 West 3rd Street Little Rock, AR 72201-1904	501-371-2640 Toll free in AR only: 1-800-282-9134 Toll free nationwide: 1-800-282-5494 Fax: 501-371-2749 E-mail: insurance.consumers@mail. state.ar.us Web site: www.state.ar.us/insurance
California	Charles Quackenbush, Insurance Commissioner Department of Insurance Executive Office 300 Capitol Mall, Suite 1500 Sacramento, CA 95814	916-493-3500 415-538-4010 San Francisco 213-897-8921 Los Angeles Toll free in CA: 1-800-927-4357 Web site: www.insurance.ca.gov

STATE INSURANCE COMMISSIONERS		
Colorado	William Airven, Commissioner Division of Insurance 1560 Broadway, Suite 850 Denver, CO 80202	303-894-7499, ext. 4311 Toll free in CO: 1-800-930-3745 TDD/TTY: 303-894-2900 Fax: 303-894-7455 Web site: www.dora.state.co.us/ Insurance
Connecticut	Raymond T. Claytor, Director Consumer Affairs Department of Insurance P.O. Box 816 Hartford, CT 06142-0816	860-297-3984 Toll free: 1-800-203-3447 Fax: 203-297-3872 Web site: www.state.ct.us/cid
Delaware	Donna Lee H. Williams, Commissioner Department of Insurance 841 Silver Lake Blvd. Dover, DE 19904	302-739-4251 Toll free in DE: 1-800-282-8611 Fax: 392-739-5380 Web site: www.state.de.us
District of Columbia	Lawrence Mirel, Commissioner District of Columbia Department of Insurance and Securities Regulation 810 First Street, NW, Suite 701 Washington, DC 20002	202-727-8000 Fax: 202-535-1196 E-mail: disr@dcgov.org
Florida	Bill Nelson, Commissioner Department of Insurance State Capitol Plaza Level Eleven Tallahassee, FL 32399-0300	850-922-3130 Toll free in FL: 1-800-342-2762 TDD toll free: 1-800-640-0886 Web site: www.doi.state.fl.us
Georgia	John Oxendine, Commissioner Insurance and Fire Safety Two Martin Luther King, Jr. Drive Atlanta, GA 30334	404-656-2070 Toll free in GA: 1-800-656-2298 TDD/TTY: 404-656-4031 Fax: 404-651-8719 Web site: www.ins.com.state.ga.us
Hawaii	Wayne Metcalf, Insurance Commis. State of Hawaii, Department of Commerce and Consumer Affairs Insurance Division 250 South King Street. 5th Floor (96813) P.O. Box 3614 Honolulu, HI 96811-3614	808-586-2790 808-586-2799 Fax: 808-586-2806 Web site: www.hawaii.gov/insurance
Idaho	Mary Hartung, Director State of Idaho Dept. of Insur. 700 West State Street P.O. Box 83720 Boise, ID 83720-0043	208-334-4250 Toll free in ID: 1-800-721-3272 Fax: 208-334-4398 Web site: www.doi.state.id.us

STATE INSURANCE COMMISSIONERS		
Illinois	Tim Cena, Office Manager and Staff Attorney Department of Insurance 100 West Randolph Street, Ste 15-100 Chicago, IL 60601	312-814-2420 Fax: 312-814-5435 Web site: www.state.il.us/ins
	Nathaniel S. Shapo, Director Department of Insurance 320 West Washington Street Springfield, IL 62767	217-782-4515 Toll free: 1-877-527-9431 (Office of Consumer Health Insurance) TDD: 217-524-4872 Fax: 217-782-5020 E-mail: director@ins.state.il.us Web site: www.state.il.us/ins/
Indiana	Sally McCarty, Commissioner Department of Insurance 311 W. Washington St., Ste. 300 Indianapolis, IN 46204-2787	317-232-2350 Toll free in IN: 1-800-622-4461 Toll free: 1-800-452-4800 (in-state senior health insurance information) Fax: 317-232-5251 Web site: www.state.in.us/idoi/
Iowa	Therese Vaughan, Commissioner State of Iowa Division of Insurance 330 Maple Street Des Moines, IA 50319	515-281-5705 Fax: 515-281-3059 Web site: www.state.ia.us/ government/com/ins/ins.htm
Kansas	Kathleen Sebelius, Commissioner Insurance Division 420 S W 9th Street Topeka, KS 66612-1678	785-296-7801 Toll free in KS: 1-800-432-2484 Fax: 785-296-2283 E-mail: ksebelius@ink.org Web site: www.ink.org/public/kid
Kentucky	George Nichols, Commissioner Department of InsuranceToll free: 1-800-595-6053 215 West Main Street Frankfort, KY 40601	502-564-3630 Fax: 502-564-1650 Web site: www/state.ky.us/ins
Louisiana	James H. Brown, Commissioner Department of Insurance 950 North Fifth Street Baton Rouge, LA 70804-9214	255-343-4834 Toll free: 1-800-259-5300 Toll free: 1-800-259-5301 Fax: 254-342-5900 Web site: www/ldi.state.la.us
Maine	Alessandro Iuppa, Superintendent Bureau of Insurance 34 State House Station Augusta, ME 04333	207-624-8475 Toll free in ME: 1-800-300-5000 TDD: 207-624-8563 Fax: 207-624-8599 Web site: www.maineinsurancereg.org

STATE INSURANCE COMMISSIONERS		
Maryland	Steven B. Larsen, Insur. Comm. Maryland Insurance Admin. 525 St. Paul Place Baltimore, MD 21202	410-468-2000 410-468-2340 (property & casualty complaints) Toll free nationwide: 1-800-492-6116 Fax: 410-468-2020 Web site: www.mia.state.ms.us
Massachu- setts	Linda Ruthardt, Commissioner Division of Insurance South Station, 5th Floor Boston, MA 02110	617-521-7794 TDD: 617-621-7490 Fax: 617-621-7772 Web site: www.state.ma.us/doi
Michigan	Frank Fitzgerald, Commissioner of Insurance Michigan Insurance Bureau 611 West Ottawa Street 2nd Floor North P.O. Box 30220 Lansing, MI 48933	517-373-0220 Toll free: 1-877-999-6442 Fax: 517-335-4978 Web site: www.cis.state.mi.us/ins

Minnesota	Gary A. LaVasseur, Deputy
	  Commissioner of Enforcement and
	  Licensing
	Department of Commerce
	133 East 7th Street
	St. Paul, MN 55101
		651-296-2488
		Toll free: 1-800-657-3602
		Fax: 651-296-4328
		E-mail: enforcement@state.mn.us
		Web site: www.commerce.state.mn.us

Mississippi	George Dale, Commissioner of Insurance Department of Insurance P.O. Box 79 Jackson, MS 39205	601-359-3569 Toll free in MS: 1-800-562-2957 Fax: 601-359-2474 Web site: www.doi.state.ms.us
Missouri	Keith Wenzel, Director Missouri Department of Insurance P.O. Box 690 301 W. High St., Room 630 Jefferson City, MO 65102	573-751-4126 575-751-2640 Toll free in MO: 1-800-726-7390 TDD/TTY: 573-526-4536 Fax: 573-751-1165 E-mail: dsprings@mail.state.mo.us Web site: www.insurance.state.mo.us
Montana	Mark O'Keefe, Commissioner Department of Insurance 840 Helena Avenue P.O. Box 4009 Helena, MT 59601	406-444-2040 Toll free in MT: 1-800-332-6148 Fax: 406-444-3497 Web site: www.state.mt.u/sao
Nebraska	L. Tim Wagner, Director Department of Insurance 941 O Street, Suite 400 Lincoln, NE 68508-3690	402-471-2201 TDD toll free: 1-800-933-7351 Fax: 402-471-4610 Web site: www.nol.org/home/NDOI
Nevada	Division of Insurance Consumer Service Section 1665 Hot Springs Road, #152 Carson City, NV 89706	775-687-7690 775-687-7650 Fax: 775-687-3937 Web site: www.doi.state.nv.us

STATE INSURANCE COMMISSIONERS		
New Hampshire	Paula Rogers, Commissioner Department of Insurance 56 Old Suncook Road Concord, NH 03301-7317	603-271-2261 Toll free in NH: 1-800-852-3416 TDD/TTY toll free in NH: 1-800-735-2964 Fax: 603-271-1406 E-mail: requests@ins.state.nh.us Web site: www.state.nh.us/insurance
New Jersey	Karen L. Suter, Acting Comm. Department of Banking & Insur. 20 West State Street P.O. Box 325 Trenton, NJ 08625	609-633-7667 Fax: 609-984-5273 Web site: http://states.naic.org/nj/NJHOMEPG.HTML
New Mexico	D.J. Leather, Superintendent Department of Insurance P.O. Box 1269 Sante Fe, NM 87504-1269	505-827-4601 Toll free in NM: 1-800-947-4722 Fax: 505-827-4734 Web site: www.nmprc.state.nm.us
New York	Consumer Services Bureau NYS Insurance Department Agency Bldg. 1-ESP Empire State Plaza Albany, NY 12257	518-474-6600 Fax: 518-474-6630 Web site: www.ins.state.ny.us
	Consumer Services Bureau NYS Insurance Department 65 Court Street #7 Buffalo, NY 14202	716-847-7618 Fax: 716-847-7925 Web site: www.ins.state.ny.us
North Carolina	James E. Long, Commissioner Department of Insurance Dobbs Building, 430 North Salisbury Street P.o. Box 26387 Raleigh, NC 27611	919-733-7349 919-733-7343 Toll free: 1-800-546-5664 Toll free: 1-800-662-7777 Fax: 919-733-6495 E-mail: bstevens@ncdoi.net Web site: www.ncdoi.net
North Dakota	Glenn Pomeroy, Insur. Comm. North Dakota Insurance Dept. 600 East Boulevard Avenue 5th Floor Bismarck, ND 58505	Toll free in ND: 1-800-247-0560 701-328-2440 TTY/TDD: 1-800-366-6888 Fax: 701-328-4880 E-mail: insurance@state.nd.us Web site: www.state.nd.us/ndins

STATE INSURANCE COMMISSIONERS

Ohio	Nancy Colley, Consumer Advocate/
	  Assistant Director
	Department of Insurance
	Office of Consumer Services
	2100 Stella Court
	Columbus, OH 43215-1067
		614-644-3378
		Toll free: 1-800-686-1526 (consumer
		  hotline)
		Toll free: 1-800-686-1527 (fraud
		  hotline)
		Toll free: 1-800-686-3745 (senior
		  hotline)
		614-644-3745
		Fax: 614-752-0740
		E-mail: nancy.colley@ins.state.oh.us
		Web site: www.state.oh.us/

Oklahoma	Carroll Fisher, Insurance Comm. Oklahoma Insurance Dept. 3814 North Santa Fe P.O. Box 53408 Oklahoma City, OK 73118	405-521-2828 Toll free in OK: 1-800-522-0071 Fax: 405-521-6652 E-mail: okinsdpt@telepath.com Web site: www.oid.state.ok.us
Oregon	Charles Nicoloff, Acting Admin. Oregon Insurance Division 350 Winter Street, NE Room 440-2 Salem, OR 97310-3883	503-947-7984 503-947-7983 Toll free in OR: 1-888-877-4894 Fax: 503-378-4351 E-mail: dcbs.insmail@state.or.us Web site: www.cbs.state.or.us/ins
Pennsylvania	Carolyn Morris, Director Bureau of Consumer Service Insurance Department 1321 Strawberry Square, 13th Floor Harrisburg, PA 17120	717-787-2317 Toll free: 1-877-881-6388 E-mail: consumer@ins.state.pa.us Web site: www.insurance.state.pa.us

Puerto Rico	Juan Antonio Garcia, Commissioner of
	  Insurance
	Office of the Commissioner of
	  Insurance
	Call Box 8330
	Fernandez Juncos Station
	Santurce, PR 00910-8330
		787-722-8686
		787-721-5858
		Fax: 787-722-4402

Rhode Island	Alfonso E. Mastrostefano, Super. Insurance Division 233 Richmond St., Suite 233 Providence, RI 02903-4233	401-222-2223 Fax: 401-222-5475
South Carolina	Ernst N. Csiszar, Director S.C. Department of Insurance Consumer Services 1612 Marion Street P.O. Box 100105 (29202-3105) Columbia, SC 29201	803-737-6180 Toll free in SC: 1-800-768-3467 Fax: 803-737-6231 E-mail: ensmmail@doe.state.sc.us Web site: www.state.sc.us/doi/

STATE INSURANCE COMMISSIONERS		
South Dakota	Darla L. Lyon, Director South Dakota Division of Insur. Department of Commerce and Regulation 118 West Capitol Pierre, SC 57501-2000	605-773-3563 Fax: 605-773-5369 E-mail: darlal@crpr1.state.sd.us Web site: www.state.sc.us/insurance

Tennessee	Anne Pope, Commissioner
	Department of Commerce and
	  Insurance
	500 James Robertson Parkway
	5th Floor
	Nashville, TN 37243-0565
		615-741-2241
		Toll free in TN: 1-800-342-4029
		  (consumer insurance services)
		Toll free in TN: 1-800-525-2816
		  (counseling for seniors)
		Fax: 615-532-5934
		Web site: www.state.tn.us/commerce

Texas	Jose Monyemayor, Commissioner of
	  Insurance
	Texas Department of Insurance
	333 Guadalupe Street (Zip 78701)
	P.O. Box 149104
	Austin, TX 78614-9104
		512-463-6169
		Toll free in TX: 1-800-252-3439 (con-
		  sumer help line)
		Fax: 512-475-2005
		Web site: www.tdi.state.tx.us

Utah	Merwin Stewart, Commissioner Department of Insurance State Office Building, Rm. 3110 Salt Lake City, UT 84114	801-538-3805 Toll free in UT: 1-800-439-3805 TDD: 801-538-3826 Fax: 801-538-3829 Web site: www.insurance.state.us.us
Vermont	Elizabeth R. Costle, Comm. Dept. of Banking, Insurance, Securities and Health Care Administration 89 Main Street Drawer 20 Montpelier, VT 05620-3101	802-828-3302 Toll free in VT: 1-800-964-1784 Fax: 802-828-3301 Web site: www.state.vt.us/bis
Virgin Islands	Maryleen Thomas, Director of Insurance Kongen's Garden #18 St. Thomas, VI 00802	340-774-7166 Fax: 340-774-9458 E-mail: cidoi001@aol.com
Virginia	Alfred W. Gross, Commissioner Bureau of Insurance State Corporation Commission P.O. Box 1157 1300 East Main Street (23219) (only for special delivery and walk-ins) Richmond, VA 23218	804-371-9967 Toll free in VA: 1-800-552-7945 TDD: 804-371-9349 Web site: www.state.va.us/scc
Washington	Deborah Senn, Commissioner of Insurance Office of the Comm. of Insur. 14th Avenue and Water Street P.O. Box 40255 Olympia, WA 98504-0255	360-753-3613 Toll free in WA: 1-800-562-6900 TDD: 360-664-3165 Fax: 360-586-3535 E-mail: inscomr@aol.com Web site: www.wa.gov/ins

STATE INSURANCE COMMISSIONERS		
West Virginia	Hanley C. Clark, Commissioner Department of Insurance 1124 Smith St., (25301) P.O. Box 50540 Charleston, WV 25305-0540	304-558-3354 Toll free in WV: 1-800-642-9004 Fax: 304-558-0412 E-mail: wvins@wvnvm.wvnet.edi Web site: www.state.wv.us/insurance
Wisconsin	Connie O'Connell, Commissioner Office of the Comm. of Insur. 121 East Wilson St., (53702) P.O. Box 7873 Madison, WI 53707-7873	608-266-0103 Toll free in WI: 1-800-236-8517 TDD/TTY toll free: 1-800-947-3529 Fax: 608-266-9935 E-mail: information@oci.state.wi.us Web site: badger.state.wi.us/ agencies/oci
Wyoming	John McBride, Commissioner Wyoming Department of Insur. Herschler Building 122 West 25th Street 3rd Floor East Cheyenne, WY 82202-0440	307-777-0401 Toll free in WY: 1-800-438-5768 Fax: 307-777-5895 E-mail: wyinsdep@state.wy.us Web site: www.state.wy.us/ ~insurancde

PLAN OF TREATMENT FOR OUTPATIENT REHABILITATION *(COMPLETE FOR INITIAL CLAIMS ONLY)*

1. PATIENT'S LAST NAME	FIRST NAME M.I.	2. PROVIDER NO.	3. HICN

4. PROVIDER NAME	5. MEDICAL RECORD NO. *(Optional)*	6. ONSET DATE	7. SOC. DATE

8. TYPE: ☐ PT ☐ OT ☐ SLP ☐ CR ☐ RT ☐ PS ☐ SN ☐ SW

9. PRIMARY DIAGNOSIS *(Pertinent Medical D.X.)*	10. TREATMENT DIAGNOSIS	11. VISITS FROM SOC.

12. PLAN OF TREATMENT FUNCTIONAL GOALS

GOALS *(Short Term)*

OUTCOME *(Long Term)*

PLAN

13. SIGNATURE *(professional establishing POC including prof. designation)*

14. FREQ/DURATION *(e.g., 3/Wk x 4 Wk.)*

I CERTIFY THE NEED FOR THESE SERVICES FURNISHED UNDER THIS PLAN OF TREATMENT AND WHILE UNDER MY CARE ☐ N/A

17. CERTIFICATION FROM   THROUGH   ☐ N/A

15. PHYSICIAN SIGNATURE   16. DATE

18. ON FILE *(Print/type physician's name)* ☐

20. INITIAL ASSESSMENT *(History, medical complications, level of function at start of care. Reason for referral)*

19. PRIOR HOSPITALIZATION FROM   TO   ☐ N/A

21. FUNCTIONAL LEVEL *(End of billing period)*   PROGRESS REPORT   ☐ CONTINUE SERVICES *OR* ☐ DC SERVICES

22. SERVICE DATES FROM   THROUGH

FORM HCFA-700 (11-91)

Appendix A-7.3. Form 700. These materials are available free of charge from HCFA at www.hcfa.gov. Any uncertainty as to whether the manual or form is still current should be resolved by contacting HCFA or the appropriate HCFA contractor.

DEPARTMENT OF HEALTH AND HUMAN SERVICES
HEALTH CARE FINANCING ADMINISTRATION

FORM APPROVED
OMB NO. 0938-0227

UPDATED PLAN OF PROGRESS FOR OUTPATIENT REHABILITATION
(Complete for Interim to Discharge Claims. Photocopy of HCFA-700 or 701 is required)

1. PATIENT'S LAST NAME	FIRST NAME	M.I.	2. PROVIDER NO.	3. HICN

4. PROVIDER NAME	5. MEDICAL RECORD NO. *(Optional)*	6. ONSET DATE	7. SOC. DATE

8. TYPE:
☐ PT ☐ OT ☐ SLP ☐ CR
☐ RT ☐ PS ☐ SN ☐ SW

9. PRIMARY DIAGNOSIS *(Pertinent Medical D.X.)* | 10. TREATMENT DIAGNOSIS | 11. VISITS FROM SOC.

12. FREQ/DURATION *(e.g., 3/Wk x 4 Wk.)*

13. CURRENT PLAN UPDATE, FUNCTIONAL GOALS *(Specify changes to goals and plan)*

GOALS *(Short Term)*

OUTCOME *(Long Term)*

PLAN

I HAVE REVIEWED THIS PLAN OF TREATMENT AND RECERTIFY A CONTINUING NEED FOR SERVICES. ☐ N/A ☐ DC

14. RECERTIFICATION
FROM   THROUGH   ☐ N/A

15. PHYSICIAN'S SIGNATURE | 16. DATE | 17. ON FILE *(Print/type physician's name)* ☐

18. REASON(S) FOR CONTINUING TREATMENT THIS BILLING PERIOD *(Clarify goals and necessity for continued skilled care)*

19. SIGNATURE *(or name of professional, including prof. designation)*	20. DATE	21. ☐ CONTINUE SERVICES *OR* ☐ DC SERVICES

22. FUNCTIONAL LEVEL *(at end of billing period - Relate your documentation to functional outcomes and list problems still present)*

23. SERVICE DATES
FROM   THROUGH

FORM HCFA-701 (11-91)

Appendix A-7.4. Form 701. These materials are available free of charge from HCFA at www.hcfa.gov. Any uncertainty as to whether the manual or form is still current should be resolved by contacting HCFA or the appropriate HCFA contractor.

Business Management Aids for the Employer

STRENGTHS

1. Location
2. Experience
3. Reputation
4. Motivated therapist
5. Stable staff
6. Atmosphere

WEAKNESSES

1. High profile competition
2. Relatively small budget
3. Small clinic (can also be a strength)
4. Minimal time to market services
5. Therapist often going many directions
6. Office isn't always "open"

OPPORTUNITIES

1. Growth potential
2. Possibility for additional contracts

3. Market need for occupational therapy services in birth to three programs in neighboring counties
4. Many marketing opportunities in neighboring communities

THREATS

1. Large facility competition
2. Change in regulations for payment of OT services in the future?
3. Large employer's potential change of group insurance to carrier in a non-participating plan
4. Continued reductions in government insurance reimbursement for OT services
5. Referral sources leaving the area

BARRIERS (to reaching full potential) – optional

1. Poor motivation to schedule physician visits, physician/marketing visits
2. Manager frequently out of the office
3. Fluctuating "in" office hours due to multi-location services

Appendix B-1.1. Sample SWOT Analysis. ©2001, Delmar, a division of Thomson Learning

ACCEPTABLE QUESTIONS	UNACCEPTABLE QUESTIONS
Have you ever used another name?	What is your maiden name?
What is your place of residence?	Do you own or rent your own home?
Are you over 18 years old?	What is your birth date?
Can you provide verification of your right to work in the U.S.?	Are you a U.S. citizen?
What languages can you speak, read or write?	Where were you born?
	What is your native tongue?
	Where were your parents born?
Can you perform the functions of this job with or without reasonable accommodation?	Do you have any physical disabilities?
How would you perform these functions?	Do you have a disability that would interfere in your ability to perform the job?
Can you meet the attendance requirements of this job?	How many days were you sick last year?
Have you ever been convicted of a felony?	Have you ever been arrested?
What skills have you acquired through military service?	When did you serve in the military?
	How were you discharged?
What professional organizations you do you belong to?	What organizations or clubs do belong to?
	What is your height and weight?
	What race are you?
	What does your spouse do?
	How many children do you have?
	How old are your children?

Appendix B-1.2. Guidelines Regarding Discriminatory Questions (Hosford-Dunn, Dunn, and Harford, 1995). ©2001, Delmar, a division of Thomson Learning

- How would you describe your clinical skills?
- What are your favorite areas of practice?
- What do you like best about being an OT/COTA/office manager, etc.?
- What do you like the least?
- Describe what expectations you have for your next job.
- Describe the qualities you would like to see in your next supervisor.
- Explain what you believe to be your strength.
- What do others see as your strength?
- What areas do you feel you need to improve?
- What have others given you constructive feedback about?
- How do you handle workplace conflict?
- Describe your reaction to constructive feedback or criticism.
- How do you feel you would meet the needs of the present opening?
- What ideas do you have about the position?
- What new areas of practice would you like to learn?
- List short and long range goals for yourself.
- How timely are you with deadlines and paperwork requirements?
- Can you perform the functions of this job with or without reasonable accommodations?

Appendix B-1.3. Appropriate Interview Questions. ©2001, Delmar, a division of Thomson Learning

MEMO

TO:

DATE: March 12, 2001

SUBJECT: New Program Justification
                Multi-Sensory Treatment Clinic

CC:

With a greater number of elementary and high school aged children requiring medication and/or suffering from Attention Deficit Disorder (ADD), and Attention Deficit Hyperactivity Disorder (ADHD), as well as all the varieties of autistic conditions prevalent today, it seems evident that an approach to helping these children learn in school would be a most valuable service to the community. The proposed program described below would meet the needs of this population by offering a program designed to address the multi-sensory needs of the child with the goal to prepare them for after school homework and daily living tasks. A tutoring service could also be implemented as well, following the treatment session. A more detailed description of the program is described below:

PROGRAM DESCRIPTION

A multi-sensory, sensory integration clinic for children and young adults who are challenged by dysfunctional sensory processing which interferes in their ability to complete school and/or work assignments. The 30-minute treatment session will be provided on a one-on-one basis. An individual program will be developed based on each participant's sensory profile. The stimulation or inhibition offered may include music, lights, textures, colors, visual, and auditory input, e.g., bubble and lava lamps, and color wheel. Comfortable lounging on a beanbag chair, hammock, or swing can further facilitate a calming atmosphere. A plastic ball pool is also available for appropriate individuals.

Following each session, the individual is required to work with their attendant, tutor, parent, or guardian for a minimum of 30 minutes to complete previously established work.

The outcome of the program will be determined by the goals(s) attainment over 3-month intervals. It is expected that an established project or assignment(s) will be completed during each quarter. Charges will be based on a 1-hour session, including one-half hour of one-on-one with a therapist, and the remainder supervised by the therapist. Charges will be _____ dollars per hour.

The program is expected to seek 5 patients per week initially, with growth potential to 10 within 6 months. Revenue for this project is identified as _____dollars per month growing to _____ dollars per month, within 1 year. Although present net profits are projected as only _____ dollars per month, it is an opportunity to create a new market niche that is valuable to the community.

In addition, the space to be used has not been well utilized in the last 6 months.

Investment for start-up equipment and supplies is approximately _____ dollars. Ongoing supplies are minimal with primary expense being OT salaries.

Because there is an occupational therapist on staff with interest in the program and she presently notes there is time in her schedule, it is an opportune time to implement this program. The program would be implemented in an off-site clinic on Jones Street, which is in a convenient location to the schools.

FUNDING

The Health and Family Services Learning Resources Program as a supplement to private and non-government insurance policies will provide funding. A program would be available to students during pre-homework times of the day such as directly after the school day.

Appendix B-2.1. New Program Justification (*continues*). ©2001, Delmar, a division of Thomson Learning

MARKETING

Marketing these new services will be done through personal contact with potential referring sources. The program will be coordinated with Health and Human Services and the Lakeside School District. These parties have both been involved in the initial discussion stages of this program and are in full support of its inception. It is recommended that development of the program and implementation of it begin for the fall term of 2002-03, coordinated with the school calendar schedule.

Appendix B-2.1 New Program Justification *(continued)*. ©2001, Delmar, a division of Thomson Learning

AGREEMENT BETWEEN _____
AND _____

_____ and _____ mutually agree to the conditions listed below:

1. _____ will provide the following services to the School District of _____:

   a. Provide occupational therapy as described in each Individualized Educational Plan for students on the assigned caseload. The services will be provided in the school at which student is enrolled.

   b. Participate in the development of IEPs for students on the assigned caseload assuring that the occupational therapy services depicted on the IEPs will be implemented accurately as identified in the established IEP.

   c. Participate in placement committee meetings for students on the assigned caseload.

   d. Complete occupational therapy reevaluations and participate in the three year reevaluation meetings for students on the assigned case load.

   e. Complete occupational therapy initial evaluations and participate in evaluation team meetings for students assigned.

   f. Request an IEP meeting and assist the IEP committee in revising a student's IEP when occupational therapy services are no longer recommended for a student.

   g. Participate in Section 504 Identification/Accommodation meetings when assigned by School Psychologist.

   h. Serve as a consultant to _____ School District on occupational therapy and assistive technology issues as well as other special education issues.

   I. Comply with all requirements and timelines related to the provision of occupational therapy in _____ Administrative Code Chapter _____, _____ School District policy.

2. _____ will maintain the appropriate documentation for students on the assigned caseload for purposes of third party reimbursement.

3. The occupational therapist designated to provide the services specified in the agreement is approved by the _____ School District. He/she will have a current _____ Department of Regulation and Licensing Occupational Therapist/Occupational Therapist Assistant certification.

4. _____ will submit a schedule to the Special Education Director identifying when services will be provided for each student on the caseload.

5. _____ will submit a log of hours to _____ on a bi-monthly basis, specifying the number of hours and the type of service provided.

6. _____ School District will pay _____ per above invoice at a rate of $_____ per hour for services rendered.

7. The agreement is effective from July 1, _____ through June 30, _____. Renewal of contract will be based on mutual agreement of both parties.

8. _____ may use the services of an occupational therapy assistant (OTA) to provide direct services to students if, a.) in _____ professional judgment, the quality of occupational therapy will not be diminished, b.) the assistant holds the appropriate _____ Department of Public Instruction license, and c.) the specific individual providing the therapy is agreed to by the _____ School District. All services provided by an Occupational Therapist for consultation and supervision of OTA will also be approved by _____ at the _____ School District.

Appendix B- 2.2. Sample Contract for OT Services with School District (*continues*). ©2001, Delmar, a division of Thomson Learning

9. The _____ School District will provide space and supplies necessary for completion of occupational therapy services as required to meet the goals stated in the IEP for each student.

10. The _____ School District will pay travel time in the amount of $_____ per hour for each visit to render OT services, participate in IEP, E-team meetings, supervise OTA, and for evaluations performed by the occupational therapist.

11. Both parties will make significant effort to coordinate IEP meetings during regular scheduled visits to _____ School District by the occupational therapist. The occupational therapist will make every effort to attend all meetings, however if scheduling conflict occurs, a conference call and/or a prior meeting with parent(s)/OTR, including documentation, will be completed.

12. _____ will schedule all therapy and evaluation times with individual classroom teacher taking into consideration the best interest of the student's educational experience.

13. _____. will provide OT services up to ____ hours per week __% FTE unless requested by school district.

_____

School District Representative/Date

_____

Facility Representative/Date

Appendix B- 2.2.   Sample Contract for OT Services with School District *(continued)*. ©2001, Delmar, a division of Thomson Learning

PROFESSIONAL GOAL SHEET AND ACTION PLAN

Employee _____

Department _____

PERFORMANCE OBJECTIVE	RESPONSIBLE PARTIES	TARGET DATE	EXPECTED OUTCOME	ACTUAL OUTCOME	INITIALS

Appendix B-4.1. Professional Goal Sheet and Action Plan. ©2001, Delmar, a division of Thomson Learning

Performance Review Form

Employee:
Date of Review:
Date of Hire:

RATING SCALE:
Always   5
Almost always (75%)   4
Usually (50%)   3
Needs improvement (25%)   2
Continues to need improvement   1*
Unacceptable (never)   0*
*will be addressed in attached goal sheet with action plan

Performance areas	Ability to perform duties of the job	Rating
Takes initiative and responsibility for duties		
Is timely in attendance to work and for appointments		
Completes paperwork requirements thoroughly and on a timely basis		
Stays on schedule, acknowledges patients if delayed		
Notifies supervisor in timely manner if unable to attend work		
Handles workload with confidence and ease		
Accepts supervision		
Follows policies and procedures		
Handles feedback positively		
Provides direction and supervision to others as needed		

Appendix B-4.2. Sample Performance Review form *(continues).* ©2001, Delmar, a division of Thomson Learning

Performance areas	Ability to perform duties of the job	Rating
Supervises co-workers and students appropriately		
Clearly communicates instructions and intentions to patients		
Implements accurate, thorough, and skilled OT		
Takes initiative to study unfamiliar treatment techniques and procedures		
Communicates effectively with patients, supervisor, and co-workers		
Resolves conflict issues appropriately		
Presents self professionally to others in dress, body language, and overt expression		
Treats patients with compassion, helps patients to feel confidence in therapy		
Accepts other duties as assigned with a positive attitude		
Additional Comments: (attach copy of goal sheet)		

Employee Signature

Manager Signature

Appendix B-4.2. Sample Performance Review form *(continued)*. ©2001, Delmar, a division of Thomson Learning

Answer the following questions with collaboration from OT staff.

1. What does your business offer that is unique to the community?

2. How do these services differ from the competition?

3. List all competitors.

4. What are the strengths of your competitors?

5. What are the weaknesses of the competition?

6. How can your business capitalize on competitor's weaknesses?

7. How can your business respond to the strengths of the competitors?

8. How can you business strengthen its market "niche"?

**Complete the following information to identify the market
for traditional and non-traditional OT services**

1. Who are the consumers?

2. What are the needs of each consumer?

3. Are the needs of the consumer being met? If not, what are the areas of need?

4. What marketing approach is most appropriate for each consumer?

5. What are the settings presently served?

6. How can these services be improved?

7. What settings could be targeted for future services and why?

8. What marketing techniques will be used to address new or underserved populations?

Appendix B-5.2. Defining the Consumer. ©2001, Delmar, a division of Thomson Learning

Complete the questions below when expanding services.

1. Who are your primary referral sources?

2. Why do they refer?

3. Are their needs being met?

4. How are they acknowledged for referrals given?

5. Who are your occasional referral sources?

6. Are their needs being met?

7. How can referrals be increased by these sources?

8. Who are the potential referral sources?

9. Why don't they refer?

10. What marketing approach is appropriate for occasional and potential referral sources?

Develop a Market Plan for a more effective approach to consumers

Marketing goals:

   1.

   2.

   3.

   4.

   5.

Marketing approach: Date to be completed by:

   1.   1.

   2.   2.

   3.   3.

   4.   4.

   5.   5.

Type of follow up to marketing:

   1.

   2.

   3.

   4.

   5.

How will effectiveness be determined?

   1.

   2.

   3.

   4.

   5.

Appendix B-5.4. Marketing Plan. ©2001, Delmar, a division of Thomson Learning

PEER REVIEW
DOCUMENTATION AUDIT

Date of audit:

Chart reviewed:

Password of reviewer:

Therapist reviewed:

DOCUMENTATION CHECKLIST:	PRESENT IN CHART:	NOT PRESENT:
Physician order prior to tx initiation, including: Physician signature		
Recertification signature at least every 30 days		
Pertinent Medical Hx		
Prior level of function		
Present level of function (for progress and d/c reports)		
Objective findings		
Objective and subjective changes for progress and d/c reports		
Functional deficits		
Functional gains (for progress and d/c reports)		
Short-term goals are measurable, functional, and lead to long term goals		
Long term goals are measurable and functional		
Rehab potential is addressed		
Home exercise program is described		
Discussion with family, caregivers, and or team members is documented		
Daily note is present for each session billed		
Entry is complete for each procedure billed		
Progress is reported a minimum of every 30 days		
Consumer response to treatment indicated		
Diagnosis is compatible with procedures and length of treatment		

Appendix B-6.1. Peer Review Form *(continues).* ©2001, Delmar, a division of Thomson Learning

DOCUMENTATION CHECKLIST:	PRESENT IN CHART:	NOT PRESENT:
Medical necessity is evidenced by:		
Frequency of tx sessions (x's/week)		
Duration of tx (minutes/tx)		
Length of tx (weeks/months)		
Reason for d/c		
Recommendations		
Future		
Instruction to pt/caregiver		

STRENGTHS OF DOCUMENTATION

1.

2.

3.

4.

ACTION PLAN FOR OMISSIONS and DEFICIENCIES

Documentation omission or error: Plan to correct deficiency:

1.

2.

3.

4.

Appendix B-6.1. Peer Review Form *(continued).* ©2001, Delmar, a division of Thomson Learning

LETTER OF MEDICAL NECESSITY

MARY

DOB: 3/25/77

DIAGNOSIS: Cerebral palsy, severe cognitive deficits

EQUIPMENT REQUESTED: Metalcraft Modular Seating System with headrest, lap tray and adjustment to current wheelchair including foot plates, calf strap

Mary is a 21 year old female who is completely nonambulatory. She is currently completing her last year in special education at her resident school district. There are plans for her to go to a specialized workshop next year. It is essential that Mary be properly positioned in her wheelchair for her to achieve her maximal potential in these settings.

Current seating components are old and worn. The back can no longer be adjusted properly causing Mary to lean backward with head back and visual attention is generally toward the ceiling. Subsequently she does not readily attend to what is directly in front of her. This will be a disadvantage toward any vocational training. Her seat does not provide adequate support and she slides forward frequently. Recommended modular seating will provide contours in both back and seat components that will provide the stability that Mary needs for optimal function.

Mary also requires that foot plates be replaced. Current foot plates do not fit the wheelchair. She will also require a calf strap to prevent legs from slipping off backwards.

Mary will also require a lap tray for her wheelchair, which will serve as both an upper extremity support and functional work surface.

Thank you for providing this necessary equipment.

_____   _____
Therapist   Date

LETTER OF MEDICAL NECESSITY

GEORGE

DOB: 1/18/43

DIAGNOSIS: Degenerative joint disease, obesity, left AKA, CHF

EQUIPMENT REQUESTED: custom oversize power wheelchair with pressure relief cushion and adjustable height armrests, oversize bedside commode

George is a 55 year old male who weighs 425 lbs. He has been a lower extremity amputee for over 30 years and suffers from painful arthritis in all joints but particularly the right knee and left shoulder. He also has a history of bilateral carpal tunnel syndrome and problems with the left rotator cuff. Moving his own weight causes much wear and tear on his joints. He also has cardiac problems. Generally he is able to transfer independently but can have flair ups of arthritic pain so severe that he struggles tremendously. He is able to perform much of his self care, light housekeeping tasks, and is an artist. Goals at this time would be to maintain function as possible through joint preservation, regular activity and range of motion exercises.

A power wheelchair is strongly recommended to accomplish the above goals. Pt will require customization to accommodate his size. The ideal wheelchair will be adjustable to allow for optimal positioning. George requires some back angle recline. Adjustable height armrests are necessary to provide upper extremity support to reduce the destructive effects of inflammation and to provide best leverage for transfer. He will also require a custom seat cushion for pressure relief as he has had incidence of skin breakdown around the coccyx from sitting.

George will also require a bedside commode to use when acute exacerbation of arthritic pain and stiffness greatly hinder his mobility.

Thank you for providing this necessary equipment.

_____
Therapist

_____
Date

Websites Mentioned in Text

Chapter 3

Chapter 6

Chapter 7

Chapter 8

Chapter 9

Other useful sites not listed in text:

www.accessunlimited.com
Access Unlimited

www.abledata.com
Able Data

www.childrenwithdisabilities.ncjrs.org
Children with Disabilities

http://clinweb2.kumc.edu/
Clinical Web Server

www.naotd.org/linklink.htm
Disability Link Sites

www.atnet.org
Assistive Technology Network

References

The American Medical Association. (2000). *Current Procedural Terminology CPT-4.* Chicago, Illinois: Author.

Angelo, Jennifer, & Smith, Roger, O. (1992). An analysis of computer-related articles in occupational therapy periodicals. *American Journal of Occupational Therapy, 47* (1): 25–29.

Bangs, Jr., & David H. (1998a). *The business planning guide: Creating a plan for success in your own business.* Chicago, Illinois: Dearborn Trade Publishing

Bangs, Jr., & David H. (1998b). *The market planning guide: Market your business, product, or service.* Chicago, Illinois: Dearborn Trade Publishing

Bauer, David G. (1995). *The "how to" grants manual.* Phoenix, Arizona: The Oryx Press and the American Council on Education.

Beaufert B. & Longest, Jr., (1990). *Management practices for health professions (Fourth Edition).* Norwalk, Connecticut: Appleton & Lang (Division of Prentice Hall).

Beck, Nancy, et al. (1996). *Managed care: An occupational therapy source book.* Bethesda, Maryland: American Occupational Therapy Association, Inc.

Christianson, Charles. (1996). Managed care: Opportunities and challenges for occupational therapy in the emerging systems of the 21st century. *American Journal of Occupational Therapy, 50:* 409–411.

Covello, Joseph A. & Hazelgren, Brian J. (1995). *The complete book of business plans: Simple steps to writing a powerful business plan.* New York, New York: Source Books, Inc.

Covey, Stephen R. et al. (1994). *First things first.* New York: Simon & Schuster.

Crispen, Cathy, & Hertfelder, Sarah D. (1990). *Private practice: Strategies for success.* Rockville, Maryland: American Occupational Therapy Association, Inc.

Downs, C. W., (2000) *Effective interviewing.* New York: Harper & Row, Inc.

Dunn, Daniel R., Harford, Earl R., & Hosford-Dunn, Holly. (1995). *Audiology business and practice management.* San Diego, California: Publishing Group, Inc.

Ellenberg, D. B. (1996). Outcomes research: The history, debate, and implications for the field of occupational therapy. *American Journal of Occupational Therapy, 50* (6): 435–441.

Fishman, Stephen. 2000. *Hiring independent contractors: The employer's legal guide.* Berkeley, California: Nolo Books.

Goleman, Daniel. (1998). *Working with emotional intelligence.* New York: Bantam Books.

Health Care Financing Administration (HCFA). (2000)a. *Medicare program integrity manual.* Maryland: United States Government.

Health Care Financing Administration (HCFA). (2000)b. *Program memorandum intermediaries/carriers.* Maryland: United States Government.

Hedman, Glenn. (1990). *Rehabilitation technology.* New York: The Hawthorne Press.

Higgins, Carol A. (1997). Outcomes measurement in home health. *American Journal of Occupational Therapy, 51*(6): 458–459.

Hillestad, Steven, G. & Berkowitz, Eric, N., (1991). *Health care marketing plans from strategy to action (Second Edition).* Maryland: Aspen Publishing.

Hosford-Dunn, Holly, Dunn, Daniel R., & Harford, Earl R. (1995). *Audiology business and practice management.* San Diego, California: Singular Publishing Group, Inc.

Hunt, S. M., McKenna, S. P., McEwan, J., Williams, J. & Papp, E. (1981). The Nottingham Health Profile: Subjective health status and medical consultations. Social Science medicine 15A, 221-229.

Jacobs, Karen, & Logigian, Martha K. (1999). *Functions of a manager in occupational therapy* (Third Edition). New Jersey: Slack, Inc.

Jeffries, Elizabeth. (1996). *The heart of leadership: Influencing by design.* Dubuque, Iowa: Kendal/Hunt Publishing Company.

Jenkins, Michael, D. (1996). *Smart starting your business in...(Titles available in all 51 states).* Oasis Press.

Jenkinson, C. (1994). *Measuring health and medical outcomes.* London: University College London Press.

Jette, A., Davies, A., Cleary, P. (1986). The functional status questionnaire (FSQ): Reliability and validity when used in primary care. *Journal of General Internal Medicine, 1*(3): 143–49.

Johnson, Alton C., & Schilly, Rockwell. (1990). *Management of hospital and health services: Strategic issues and performance* (Third Edition). C. V. Mosby Company.

Kieserman, Robert. (1993). *Starting or expanding a private practice in the changing health care environment.* (Unpublished Manuscript.) Therapy Practice Management.

Kirschner, Celeste, G., et al. (2000). *Current procedural terminology.* Chicago, Illinois: American Medical Association.

Kishel & Kishel. (1993). *How to start, run, and stay in business.* New York, New York: J. Wiley & Sons Publication.

Lloyd-Jones, Joseph & Simyar, Farhad. (1998). *Strategic management in the health care sector toward the year 2000.* New Jersey: Prentice-Hall.

Lore, Nicholas. (1999). *The pathfinder: How to change your career for a lifetime of satisfaction and success.* New York: Simon and Schuster.

Mayhan, Y. D. (1994). *The importance of outcomes measurement in managed care.* Administration and Management Special Interest Section Newsletter, 10(4), 2–4.

New South Wales Health Department. (1992). The NSW health outcomes program. *New South Wales Public Health Bulletin, 3*(12): 135.

Nulman, Phillip R. (1996). *Start-up marketing: An entrepreneur's guide to advertising, marketing and promoting your business.* Carrer Press.

O'Connor, Sheila (2000). OTs and office ergonomics consulting. *OT Practice. 5* (10): 12–17.

Pinson, Linda & Jinnett, Jerry. (1996). *The anatomy of a business plan.* Chicago, Illinois: Dearborn Trade Publishing.

Przybylski, B. R., Dumont, E. D., Watkins, M. E., Warren, S. A., Beaulne, A. P., Lier, D. A. (1996). Outcomes of enhanced physical and occupational therapy service in a nursing home setting. *Archives of Physical Medicine and Rehabilitation, 77*(6), 554–61.

Schultz & Johnson. (1990). *Management of hospital and health services.* St. Louis, MO: Mosby.

Solomon, R. (1991). *Clinical practice management.* Aspen Publishing.

Thomson, L. K., & Foto, M. (1995). Elements of clinical documentation. *American Journal of Occupational Therapy. 49*(10): 1032–1035.

Velozo, C. A., Magalhaes, L., Pan, A., & Leiter, P. (1995). Differences in functional scale discrimination at admission and discharge: Rasch analysis of the Level of Rehabilitation Scale-III (LORS-III). *Archives of Physical Medicine and Rehabilitation. 76*(8), 705–712.

Ware, J. E. (2000). SF-36 Health Survey Update. *Spine, 25*(24): 3130–3139.

Ware, J. E. & Sherbourne. (1992). *SF-36 Health Survey.* Boston, MA:The Health Institute.

Recommended Readings

The American Occupational Therapy Association. *The occupational therapy manager (1995).* Rockville, Maryland: Author.

Bumphrey, Eileen. (1995). *Community practice: A text for occupational therapy and others involved in community care.* New Jersey: Prentice Hall/Harvester Wheatsheaf.

De Clive-Lowe, S. (1996). Outcome measurement, cost-effective and clinical audit: The importance of standardized assessment to occupational therapists in meeting these new demands. *British Journal of Occupational Therapy, 59*(8): 357–362.

Eklund, M. (1999). Outcome of occupational therapy in a psychiatric day care unit for long-term mentally ill patients. *Occupational Therapy in Mental Health, 14* (4): 21–45.

Dobrzykowski, Edward A., Jr. & Leiberman, Deborah. (2000). Outcomes management: Getting started. *OT Practice, 5*: 10, p. CE-1–CE-7.

Fawcett, L. C., & Strickland, L. R. (1998). Accountability and competence: Occupational therapy practitioner perceptions. *American Journal of Occupational Therapy, 52* (9): 737–743.

Feuerstein, M., Burrell L.M., Miller V.I., Lincoln, A., Huang, G.D., Berger, R. (1999). Clinical Management of Carpal Tunnel Syndrome: A 12-Year Review of Outcomes. *American Journal of Industrial Medicine. 35* (3): 232-245.

Functional Independence Measure (FIM). Buffalo, NY: Uniform Data Systems for Medical Rehabilitation.

Hunt, S. M., McKenna, S. P., McEwan, J., Williams, J. & Papp, E. (1981). The Nottingham Health Profile: Subjective health status and medical consultations. Social Science medicine 15A, 221-229.

Jette, Davis, Cleary, 96. The functional status questionnaire (FSQ): Reliability and validity when used in primary care. *Journal of General Internal Medicine, 1*(3): 143–49.

Jinnett, Jerry & Pinson, Linda. (1996). *Target marketing: researching, reaching and retaining your market.* Upstart Publishing Company.

Kaplan, Kathy L. & Ostro, Patricia C. (1987). *Occupational therapy and mental health: a guide to outcomes research.* Rockville, Maryland: American Occupational Therapy Association, Inc.

Long, A. F. (1995). Clarifying and identifying the desired outcomes of an intervention: The case of stroke *Outcomes Briefing, 5*: 10–12.

Long, A. F. & Fairfield, G. (1996). Confusion of levels in monitoring outcomes and/or process, *Lancet, 347*(9015): 1572.

McCollum, H. F., Jr., & Minders, J. M. (1984). *Hearing aid dispensing practice.* Danville, Illinois: Interstate Printers and Publishers.

Nelson Bolles, Richard (1999). *What color is your parachute? A practical manual for job hunters and career changes.* Berkeley, California: Ten Speed Press.

McDonough, Andrew L., Saidoff, David C. (1997). *Critical pathways and therapeutic intervention upper extremities.* St. Louis, MO: Mosby.

Schaughnessy, et al., 95. *Medicare OASIS.* Federal Register, Vol 64.

Scull, D. (1997). *An outcome measure for adult mental health: An evaluation study of the canadian occupational performance measure (COPM) for adult mental health.* Undergraduate Honours Theses, University of Wales. Cardiff.

Steeden, B. (1994). Occupational therapy guidelines for client-centered practice and canadian occupational performance measure: Book Review. British *Journal of Occupational Therapy, 57*, 23.

Toomey, M., Nicholson, D. Carswell, A. (1995). The clinical utility of canadian occupational performance measure. *Canadian Journal of Occupational Therapy, 62*, 242–249.

Ware, J. E. & Sherbourne. (1992). *SF-36 Health Survey.* Boston, MA:The Health Institute.

Waters, D. (1995). Recovering from a depressive episode using the Canadian occupational performance measure. *Canadian Journal of Occupational Therapy, 62*, 278–282.

Index

DATE DUE